Suicide in Intersex, Trans, and Other Sex and/or Gender Diverse Groups

A Health Professional's Guide

Suicide in Intersex, Trans, and Other Sex and/or Gender Diverse Groups

A Health Professional's Guide

Tracie O'Keefe

About Dr Tracie O'Keefe, DCH, BHSc, ND

Tracie is a sex researcher, teacher and therapist, clinical psycho-therapist, clinical hypnotherapist, counsellor, clinical supervisor, naturopath, medical nutritionist, medical herbalist, and Director of the Australian Health and Education Centre (AHEC) in Sydney, Australia. An intersex and trans woman, Tracie was born hypogonadal with a mild insensitivity to androgens but was classified as transsexual. She was forced to live for the first 15 years of her life as male against her will and then began transitioning to living as female at 15 years old. She had to battle with clinicians who were against her transition.

Tracie has worked in the sex and/or gender diverse community since being at college in 1970. She has been in private practice since 1994 at the London Medical Centre in the UK before becoming the full-time director of AHEC in 2001. In clinical practice, she has seen more than three thousand patients from sex and/or gender diverse groups as well as encountering thousands more in the community.

Tracie holds a degree in complementary medicine, a degree in clinical hypnotherapy, a post-graduate advanced diploma in psychotherapy and hypnosis, and a doctorate in clinical hypnotherapy (DCH). She is a registered mental health professional and member of the College of Psychotherapy of the Psychotherapy and Counselling Federation of Australia (PACFA), a member of the Australian Society of Sex Educators, Researchers and Therapists (ASSERT, NSW), a member of the Australian Hypnotherapists Association (AHA) and a member of the Australian Naturopathic Practitioners Association (ANPA). Apart from being a researcher, writer, teacher and clinician, she has spent decades as a political lobbyist and advocate for the human rights of sex and/or gender diverse people.

She is the co-founder of Sex and Gender Education (SAGE), Australia, a campaign group that lobbies for the rights of sex and/or gender diverse people.

Dedication

This book is dedicated to all those people from sex and/ or gender diverse groups throughout the world who have struggled with suicide; the ones who have died and the ones who chose to live. This work is for you. Know that you did not die or live in vain but rest in our thoughts. It is also dedicated to all those healthcare professionals who daily reach out to help and support our community, listen to what we say and speak publicly in our defence when we are attacked.

Finally, I dedicate this book to my friends and colleagues at Sex and Gender Education Australia (SAGE), as it is written as part of SAGE's outreach into the world to improve the lives and rights of sex and/or gender diverse groups of people.

About Sex And Gender Education (SAGE) (Australia)

SAGE campaigns for the rights and respectful dignity of sex and/ or gender diverse (SGD) groups of people in Australia on the issues affecting their everyday lives and distributes information relating to the quality of their lives.

Sex and/or gender diverse groups of people are made up of many differing populations including people who are intersex, androgynous, sex diverse, transexed, transsexual, transgendered, without sex and gender identity, crossdressers and people with culturally-specific sex and gender differences.

They are people who experience variations in physical presentation and social behaviour that are other than stereotypically male or female. Each group may have its own physical, psychological, social, legal and political issues that may not necessarily relate to any of the other groups.

SAGE as a collective has been in existence since 2001 and has contributed to several changes in law and policy in Australia that benefit SGD groups of people. An informal network of people, it is an initiative that was initially funded by community contributions and later by O'Keefe & Fox Industries Pty Ltd.

This project grew out of the work of SAGE and the need to offer health professionals guidance in helping people from SGD groups struggling with or contemplating suicide.

We honour all who have and do engage with SAGE to promote human rights for SGD groups.

"The wound is the place where the light enters you".
                                          – Rumi

Disclaimer:

This book is designed to provide general information only for health professionals who treat or plan to treat clients from sex and/or gender diverse groups of people. This information is provided and sold with the knowledge that the publisher and author do not offer any medical, legal, financial or other professional advice. In the case of a need for any such expertise, consult with the appropriate professional. This book does not contain all information available on the subject.

This book has not been created to be specific to any individuals' or organisations' situation or needs. Every effort has been made to make this book as accurate as possible. However, there may be typographical and/or content errors. Therefore, this book should serve only as a general guide and not as the ultimate source of subject information.

The examples stated in the book are not intended to represent or guarantee that anyone will achieve the same or similar results. Each individual's success depends on their background, dedication, desire and motivation.

Any and all information contained in this book or any related materials are not intended to take the place of medical advice from a healthcare professional. Any action taken based on the contents found in this book or related materials is to be used at the sole discretion and sole liability of the reader.

Under no circumstances, including, but not limited to, negligence, shall the author or O'Keefe & Fox Industries Pty Ltd be liable for any special or consequential damages that result from the use of, or the inability to use, the book and related materials in this book, even if O'Keefe & Fox Industries Pty Ltd or an O'Keefe & Fox Industries Pty Ltd authorised representative has been advised of the possibility of such damages.

This book contains information that might be dated and is intended only to educate and entertain. The author and publisher shall have no liability or responsibility to any person or entity regarding any loss or damage incurred, or alleged to have incurred, directly or indirectly, by the information contained in this book.

Published by Australian Health & Education Centre
An imprint of O'Keefe & Fox Industries Pty Ltd
Suite 207, 410 Elizabeth Street, Surry Hills, NSW 2010, Australia
Website: www.healtheducationcentre.com

International wholesale enquiries through Ingram.

Copyediting: Sarah Chalmers
Cover design by Aleksandar Novovic
Text layout: Kassandra Marsh: www.lakazdi.com

ISBN: 978-0-9875109-5-2

Warning

This book may contain highly disturbing, graphic and emotive material around death and the threat of death. It refers to those who have died. If you are triggered by traumatic material and reference to deceased persons, this work may not be for you. It may contain people from your community who have passed. If you commence reading, be aware such material can ignite or reignite trauma. If you find yourself in that position, immediately seek professional help.

In reading this book, you will be taking a deep dive into the world of sex and/or gender diverse groups of people, and this may severely and unapologetically challenge your existing beliefs.

Table of Contents

Acknowledgements

I want to acknowledge the Gadigal people of the Eora Nation whose land I rest upon while carrying out this research and project. I respect your elders past, present and emerging.

I want to thank all those people, living and deceased, who have taken part in the SAGE project over the past twenty years, fought legal cases, lobbied, marched and petitioned for human rights for sex and/or gender diverse (SGD) groups of people. Your efforts and participation are a testament to human survival and dignity.

I also acknowledge the healthcare professionals who have worked so hard for SGD groups of people for over 100 years whose work and integrity we rest upon. Some of them have had their careers threatened and even ruined for taking up the baton to advocate on behalf of SGD groups.

I want to acknowledge those campaigners, clinicians and researchers who came before me and laid the foundations of knowledge and privilege that allow us to carry out this work now.

I am especially grateful for the smart and kind people who reached out to help me personally and professionally at times of need during my own life and career.

To the people who rallied, marched, campaigned, suffered discrimination, got beaten and died in the fight for SGD equality—your story is not lost, and it is a stepping stone on which we tread to the future.

Thank you to the people who contributed their stories to

this work which shows people from SGD groups that they can overcome suicide and go on to lead meaningful and rewarding lives. Standing up and being named is brave in a world that is often hostile towards you. This is a proud act of education and political importance.

A big thank you to my wonderful wife Katrina Fox, who has tirelessly worked away on my and SAGE's behalf for nearly 20 years, dotting the i's, crossing the t's, managing the production of this book and my work in general.

My gratitude also goes to my assistant Rosalie Vinluan, who backs me up in my day-to-day practice and allows the machinery of providing clinical care to happen.

Thank you to Sarah Chalmers for early copyediting of the book.

I am immensely grateful to Australian geneticist Professor Jenny Graves for providing indepth feedback on the chapter on sex diversity.

I wish to acknowledge my own privilege of having food, a home, education and meaningful employment, which has been possible due to the legal and social in-roads of other campaigners who helped make that possible. For many people from SGD groups in the world today these privileges are still not available.

Introduction

Suicide, attempted suicide and suicidal thoughts, particularly in sex and/or gender diverse (SGD) groups, are frequently not discussed or are ignored by healthcare practitioners. It can frighten us as we are often not trained on how to guide such clients. It is ignored most of the time by politicians, policy-makers and the healthcare systems that are designed to treat acute disease rather than facilitate well-being. A client being from a SGD group complicates the incidence of suicide, and healthcare workers can find themselves out of their depths.

Suicide hits to the heart of our own sense of vulnerability as human beings and professionals. It is when, in the face of adversity, we feel overwhelmed, out of control, cornered by life, deserted by good fortune and unable to forge our own destiny. Feeling powerless, we can be left with the option of ending life itself as a final act of control.

The obsession of those who seek to erase SGD groups of people is fuelled by ignorance, hate and persecution in order to bolster the oppressor's own self-importance. When politicians use these populations as political footballs by saying they do not believe in intersex, sex and/or gender diversity or that sex markers should never be changed on birth certificates, they are pursuing hate speech.

So, people from SGD groups can be left with a searing shame, guilt and hopelessness around our existence. The constant framing of us as an offensive aberration is scorched into our minds. When you grow up with a backdrop of these relentless social and political attacks, it can induce an underlying fear of life, safety and any future hope.

On top of that our experiences are appropriated and retold incorrectly by others. The medical profession has described us as nature's mistake and has forced us into being classified as a pathology before we could get the medical help we need. Just as violent may be the enforcement of medical intervention on our bodies and minds without our permission as children in an unquantified and unproven quest to 'normalise' us.

Added to this is the appropriation of our SGD narrative by those who speak for us instead of asking us to speak ourselves. Creationists, uneducated health professionals, biased academics and radical right-wing groups promote prejudice against us, justifying their views by claiming we are delusional and a danger to others.

So, this lack of acceptance of our place at the table of life and the conversation around our own existence seeks to erase us from the human equation. It is driven mainly by patriarchy, misogyny, misandry, sexism and genderism from different camps with different grievances in different conversations.

This oppression and exclusion are what underlies all intersex, trans and SGD phobias. It is fear-based aggression that seeks to control, isolate and eliminate SGD groups of people. People from SGD groups become weary and exhausted from a battle not of their making. They inherit the oppression intergenerationally and learn to live at an early age from a place of fear. When minority stressors become over-bearing, we can find suicidal thoughts a relief from those attacks.

Socially there is normally a buffer that can stop this progression to suicide happening, in the form of support from family and social association. But, and this is a very large and relevant but, many people from SGD groups have been rejected by their families and society and have no or little social support. In that isolation, they may have no support from people who are similar to them. They flounder in a hostile situation and mental desolation with feelings of abandonment to the point that suicide can appear the better option.

This book is a conversation around how healthcare professionals can offer constructive help to people from SGD groups who have become suicidal. It considers how to set up and operate suicide prevention interventions. A large part of that education is to understand the sociological circumstances in which those suicidal thoughts arise. Without that in-depth knowledge, any intervention runs the risk of being prescriptively inauthentic, patronising and ineffective.

There were campaigning interruptions to this three-year project as the right-wing and religious groups tried to introduce laws into Australia that exclude SGD groups from education, housing, medicine and social spaces. The battle for equal rights never stops so we always have to be vigilant and active in creating and maintaining civil rights.

This project was undertaken as a social welfare exercise in the face of increasing numbers of suicides of people from SGD groups throughout the world. It is as much a sociological and political work as it is clinical. Like any project, the outcome is shaped by the discoveries made during the investigation, and the work takes on a shape of its own to tell its story. It is an international story that sources experiences from around the world, so the principles and suggestions offered can apply to all cultures. It is a work to help you, the healthcare professional, build and improve your competency and confidence in working in suicide rescue and prevention with SGD groups of people.

How to use this book
This book does not seek to be an authoritative work, medical directory or academically definitive text. It is humbly written to progressively and sequentially educate you as a healthcare professional in the area of suicide prevention for SGD groups of

people. Regardless of whether you are a sexologist, researcher, psychotherapist, counsellor, psychologist, psychiatrist, nurse, general physician, naturopath, social worker or project manager, it can help you to evolve your clinical skills.

To get the best from this book, approach it with an open mind, as you just might learn a great deal. At times, you will be challenged by the debate—as you should be—so rise to the challenge and continue to learn. As healthcare professionals, we are all trained from the worldview of our own doctrines that can lead us to professional myopia which we must look beyond.

This work is meant to challenge and change the way you practise, so allow that process to happen. Allow that you may gain greater knowledge and skills for helping suicide prevention in the highly disadvantaged and oppressed SGD populations. As healthcare professionals, each new piece of information we encounter during our career is not only meant to change us professionally but also as a person.

There are themes that I revisit again and again throughout the book from different perspectives to help you gain new understandings. While as healthcare professionals we seek to practise from an ethical perspective, ethics are driven by politics, power and trading favours. The ethics of today are invariably the historical curiosities of tomorrow, so as practitioners, the true compass we are wise to follow is our intellect. Enjoy your growing experience and increasing skills to help people from SGD groups to overcome suicide.

"From the smallest acorn, the largest oak tree can grow".

The research
The research for this work is sourced from many areas including academic studies, medical and psychological databases, the media, grey literature, biographies and self-reporting. This also includes documentaries and videos.

Academic studies, while giving us considerable wide-ranging information from different cultures and institutions, are often subject to the five-year rule where studies older than five years are considered outdated. However, the subject matter we deal with has a low level of published studies and suffers from a poor level of funding so I include older studies that are still relevant.

Databases tend to publish institutional generated studies that often target a very small number or phenomenon. Using such studies alone can give a profoundly distorted perspective as they generally ignore a large number of wild variables, causing inaccurate research blindness.

I include media reporting as evidence of sociological activity. Academic and clinical studies frequently ignore media reporting, citing it as unreliable. It is true that media reporting can lack the veracity of index-linked studies. However, en masse, it does give us evidence of social phenomena by its sheer volume.

Grey literature provides further evidence of social activity, politics, ethics and human interactions. More than that, it gives us traces of individual and group footprints, activity and history.

In a work that deals with subjective human experience, thoughts and action, it is paramount that we include qualitative first-person reporting, including biographies of people who have faced sex and gender diverse issues and suicide. What they said, what happened to them and how they reacted to their life situations is enlightening.

In this work, I have abandoned using pseudonyms and all contributors use their own first name, except when relating my own cases. Much of the general research dismisses real name reporting, but it gives authentic histories and helps to dispel public shame and guilt about SGD groups' life experience and suicide.

Finally, as someone who has spent over fifty years in SGD community groups, twenty-four years in voluntary work and twenty-seven years in private clinical practice, seeing over three thousand patients from SGD groups, I break the fourth wall at times to offer my personal and professional opinions of people who have faced suicide in our community.

The referencing at the end of each chapter is not just to support the concepts I offer but also so that readers can pursue their own education and investigation on this subject. Sex and gender diversity is a large subject in a small niche of healthcare.

To gain a wide perspective on this subject, we must study the politics of everyday medicine, what the public will allow and how they behave towards SGD groups.

Some references will be eternal and some may be dated by the time of publication so you should be vigilant in searching for the current information related to the dialogue.

The language used in this book

Language, descriptions and self-descriptions change constantly in the process of social evolution and even at times devolution. It is largely out of the power of the few and in the hands of the many.

The words used here to describe people are not set in concrete or authoritative and neither do I own them. They are taken from common usage and used with intentional respect.

Those words and descriptions will change in time culturally so I beseech the reader to consider them within the context of the work and not as a judgment or reflection upon anyone's existence or identity.

Chapter 1:
What Many Sex and/or Gender Diverse People Experience Every Day

I start this work purposefully real. It is important that you understand the pressures that rest upon the shoulders of people from sex and/or gender diverse (SGD) groups who are driven towards suicide. After 50 years of working with SGD groups of people, this book is the most disturbing I have ever written. If you are triggered by trauma, do not read it.

This book highlights the seriousness of suicide in SGD groups and possible solutions. Ask yourself: Why would so many people from these populations think about, attempt and complete suicide?

The answer to this will become clear as I invite you to walk a mile in the shoes of such people for a window into their experience. You will only ever understand what this population faces when you begin to consider them within the larger social context in which they live.

If you look different, somewhere between male or female, are female with male characteristics or male with female characteristics, you can become hunted by people looking for victims. They are out there: bigots, sexists, genderists, hatemongers, trolls, religious zealots, fascists, indignant moralists, people seeking significance by harassing others and ones who mock you to try and make themselves look clever and strong. They are unkind, unreasonable, irreverent of the law, care not about social opinions and are or become psychopathic towards you in encounters. Sometimes they may even have been you, unless you have always checked yourself, your privilege and your humanity.

You may have forgotten you were or could have been them, but now is the time to reflect and consider new perspectives.

Social psychology teaches us that persecutors do not just come in ones or twos alone but from groups that infest social opinion, the law and crowds. They become the hunters and SGD groups become their prey in the crusade for a strictly male and female worldview. Should you be outside their version of a proper human being, they make it their mission to damage you and ultimately eliminate you.

When they inflict this damage, you can become fearful, unsure of yourself; the candle of hope can disappear from your eyes and after repeated exposure to that danger, you just may begin to believe that you are not deserving.

Collison (2018) reports that, in Africa, children with ambiguous genitalia, who are obviously intersexed, are frequently murdered at birth. In 2015, Nunchi Theriso (not their real name), an intersex activist, carried out a series of interviews with traditional healers, birth attendants, midwives and mothers of intersex children. It seems in some cultures the birth of an intersex child is seen as a bad omen, a curse on the family and the perceived result of witchcraft.

According to Collison, the South African Human Rights Commission reports that 70% of the population and 50% of women in that country consult traditional healers. It is therefore highly likely that under the guise of traditional healing practices, mass infanticide of intersex children is carried out to rid the families of what they see as a curse. The deaths or incidences of intersex are not reported, the children are buried and the families do not talk about what happened. Often, the mother is never told her child was intersex, just that the infant died at birth or was stillborn, and she is instructed not to talk about it.

Of the 90 traditional birth attendants' interviewed, Collison reports, 88 said they had disposed of intersex infants.

Their birth is seen as a sign that the ancestors are displeased. In response, the baby can be strangled, have its neck broken, be bashed on rocks, thrown into the river or fed to wild animals.

An estimated 150,000 teenagers in the USA identified at school as transgender (The Williams Institute, 2017). Some were intersex, others transitioning, gender fluid, more rarely androgynous, and others identified as gender queer. Some schools accommodate those children but, in a climate of minority victimisation, many do not. The situation is the same in many countries, with children having to be relocated to different schools and sometimes whole families needing to uproot from their community and move away to try and avoid harassment, bullying and physical and psychological danger to those children and to other members of the family.

Some children are out about their transitioned or intersex status at school, but others keep the fact that they are intersex or have transitioned from their peers and the local community for fear of victimisation. They can be shamed in so many different ways by other children and teachers, and excluded from many activities.

Parents of other students at times engage in campaigns to have SGD students removed from schools, citing them as being against god, perverted, mentally deranged and a danger to their own children. Children as young as four can be subjected to communications that say they are wrong, unworthy, dangerous, possessed by the devil, mentally ill and unwanted.

Georgie Stone, an Australian child, was seven years old when she transitioned at school from a little boy to a female student, at which point she had to face the bathroom issue (Stark, 2017). She dressed as a girl, went to school as a girl and asked to be addressed as female but was not allowed to use the girls' facilities at school. She said, "I just remember them jeering at me." She encountered daily bullying and going to the bathroom was a battleground. The principal told Stone's mother that allowing her to use the girls' facilities would confuse other children and cause resistance among the parents.

At 16, Stone remembered an incident when she was nine years old in the boys' changing rooms, in a girls' bathing costume with long hair. She recalled, "I just remember them jeering at me, making fun of me, shouting at me, saying, 'What's a girl doing in the male change rooms?' It was awful. I ran out half-dressed, crying my eyes out." She got changed behind a tree for the rest of the term before her parents, worried about her safety, found a different, more accepting school for her. Many children in different countries face the same issues because of adults' failure to protect SGD students. The shaming and bullying can scar a child for life and undermine their sense of being worthy to live in this world.

The Age (Jacks, 2019) newspaper in Melbourne reported the experiences of Simona Castricum, a transgender architect and Melbourne University academic. She told how she could not commute on the trains to work due to fearing for her personal safety. She had been spat on, sexually assaulted, verbally abused and intimidated by people who claimed to have been too disgusted to sit next to her; she believed this was because of her trans status.

Castricum said that when she got into rail carriages, she had to scan around her to see who the least dangerous person might be to sit next to. Castricum's every journey on public transport was a risk. Eventually, she had to travel around the city by taxi or Uber to be safe. At the time of reporting, Melbourne was rated one of the safest cities in the world.

Somewhere among the bottom of the social pecking order of sex, race, economics, class, religion, disabilities, creed and intellect, lies the basement of expectations, which is frequently people who are publicly known to be from SGD groups. Here I am not talking about the wealthy, famous, privileged and successful among us, although they suffer prejudices too, but about the average person from SGD groups who rides the subway and endures the stares of others.

The runner Caster Semenya, born intersex and raised as a female, endured years of harassment from the press as she won races (Farquhar, 2009). Her medical records were unceremoniously and illegally released to the press, without her permission, by members of the International Association of Athletics Federations (IAAF), when her competitors complained about her victories. Born with a form of complete Androgen Insensitivity Syndrome (AIS), with XY chromosomes, she had a vagina, no womb or ovaries, and small internal testes.

Semenya was hounded by the world's press. What people failed to understand, however, is that people born with AIS have little advantage in building muscle over other athletes. Androgens alone are ineffective in helping people build those muscles because you build muscle by repetition of action and the work you do on building your body's strength and endurance. If you have AIS, the only way to compete in sport is to train harder than other competitors to build muscle; you are advantaged by your performance and dedication alone.

If you have AIS, you are largely or partly insensitive to testosterone's muscle-building effects. There are many women who have high androgen levels but flaccid and ineffective muscles because they do not exercise regularly or train as an athlete.

Decades earlier, Maria José Martínez-Patiño (2005), a Spanish female hurdler, was banned in 1986 for competing as a female athlete and stripped of all her medals when she failed a genetic test that revealed she had complete AIS. She was shamed publicly as a fraud. She had been due to compete in the 1988 Olympics, but the opportunity was taken away from her. Martínez-Patiño also lost her athletics scholarship and was lambasted in the press. All her life, she had lived as and been treated as female. She was unaware she had the intersex condition until the sporting genetics test.

Martínez-Patiño fought for the restoration of her IAAF

license. She appealed to Juan Carlos, the King of Spain, Prince Albert of Monaco and Juan Antonio Samaranch, President of the IAAF.

After three years, she managed to have her license reinstated, and she competed in the 1992 Olympics. Martínez-Patiño has been very clear that she is legally, and as far as she is concerned, female, even though she has 46 XY chromosomes. The case caused the IAAF (now called World Athletics) to review its policy on genetic testing; however, it is now, in 2021, in the middle of a new controversy regarding how to differentiate between male or female, intersex and trans people competing. Athletes from SGD groups still run the risk of being disqualified and humiliated in the press.

The British journalist, interviewer and entertainer Piers Morgan is well known for making transphobic, bullying comments in front of millions of TV viewers and on Twitter. He claimed that gender fluid people were damaging society, stating, "Where I've got a problem is this whole, opting out of gender. Being gender-fluid. Waking up one day and thinking you want to be whatever you feel like. Is that not damaging to society, if we allow everyone to self-identify however the hell they like?" (Duffy, 2018a).

He said non-binary children are "a contagion", questioned the numbers of trans people who attempt suicide due to bullying, and claimed that identifying as non-binary is "a massive new fad" (Jackman, 2017). Insensitive, ill-informed comments like these get broadcasted to millions of people and panic parents of such children, increasing the level of fear and anxiety about the safety of their children, who are already struggling with being in a minority.

Children are extremely sensitive to messages posited as public opinion, which can lead to internalised depression and suicide. If it is illegal to advertise cigarettes and alcohol to children because they are sensitive to viewing material, does it then not follow that what they view on family entertainment during the daytime will also affect them?

The Rainbow Rights Watch, an Australian campaigning group, reported that around 7,000 articles referring to trans people were published in the Australian media in 2016–2017, with a large majority being negative (Berkovic, 2019). They complained to the Press Council and the NSW Civil Administration Tribunal (NCAT) that, in reporting stories, journalists used a person's trans status when it was not relevant to the story in order to sensationalise the news. NCAT referred the complaint on to the Antidiscrimination Board. The Press Council did uphold two complaints against *The Daily Mail* and *nine.com.au* that they used a person's trans status in a story about manslaughter when it was not relevant to the case.

At the time of writing, Australia does not have a policy on how a person's intersex or trans status should be handled in the media. The Rainbow Rights Watch's research made clear that currently, in many cases, the topic was being handled negatively on purpose. This is traditionally the case in almost all countries, particularly when the right-wing media seek sensationalism by creating victimisation. The media gets away with doing this to trans people in ways that they would not when reporting on women's, race or religious issues. This can give the public the impression that SGD groups are unbalanced, troublemaking and undesirable people, which makes SGD groups feel more unsafe in public.

Politicians, celebrities and journalists looking for the limelight relish controversial issues. The more controversial the issue, the better the publicity, and SGD issues can guarantee publicity. SGD issues can easily be framed to be controversial, and such opportunists do not have to believe what they say, as their aim is to create clickbait and dominate the media conversation, selling advertising spots. Often, they are speaking from absolute ignorance, but as Adolf Hitler paraphrased in *Mein Kampf* (Hitler, 1992): If you tell a big enough lie and tell it often enough, it will be believed.

Stephanie McCarthy, a 43-year-old transgender woman, suffered a fractured eye socket after being attacked and beaten by a young man outside a pub in Newtown, Sydney in 2015, for no other reason than being trans (Visentin, 2015). What was unusual about this case was that the area is designated as a LGBTIQ-friendly area, known locally as a Safe Space.

The man seemed to be under the influence of drugs and alcohol and began by pulling her hair. There is an assumption that because you are recognised as trans, you can be an object of ridicule and amusement. You can be placed in a position where ordinary social rules are suspended when it comes to your peace and safety. During the altercation, the perpetrator jumped up on a table to unleash a tirade of transphobic abuse. Yet he was sentenced only to 150 hours of community service and an 18-month good behaviour bond. He was also convicted of cannabis possession.

BBC News (Paris Transgender Woman 'Humiliated' at Protest, 2019) reported a trans woman being attacked by a crowd of Algerian protesters in Paris as she tried to go down into the Paris Metro, for no other reason than how she appeared. Their extremist views caused them to assume that they had the right to mock, shame and physically assault her in broad daylight, in public, in front of cameras. They shouted at her that she was a man so she could not pass. Such attacks are an everyday occurrence throughout the world.

The problem with these kinds of cases is that they do not require the perpetrator to learn anything, so they continue to see trans people as the enemy. Australian schools and schools in many other countries are not teaching human rights in relation to people from SGD groups. In fact, the large majority are not teaching anything around sex and gender diversity but only stereotypical, heteronormative sexism. This means young people come out of school having been indoctrinated with the idea that people from SGD groups are weird and not the norm or equal to them. Many schools of religious faith have embargos on ever teaching anything about intersex, trans or gay issues, so those students in particular are susceptible to the messages of extreme right-wing prophets.

Za'hair Martinez, a trans man living in Pittsburgh, was beaten early in the morning at his local 7-Eleven store (Sosin, 2018). He had previously moved from St. Augustine, Florida, four years earlier because his family did not accept him, and he sought a more accepting, welcoming and safe community for trans men. The area was known as an LGBTIQ-friendly area. The incident started with him being heckled and mistaken for an effeminate gay man. "A lot of people mistake me for a gay male," Martinez said. The perpetrators shouted "Faggot!" at him. Another woman threatened to throw hot coffee in his face, to which he responded, "If you throw coffee on me, then that's an issue."

The woman threw the coffee in his eyes and was then joined by a man who started to punch him. Five people then started to punch and kick Martinez and he said he heard someone shout "That's a female!" as they were kicking him. The attack lasted ten minutes but no one, including the 7-Eleven staff, called the police or emergency services. Eventually, he found someone outside who drove him to the hospital where he received stitches on his face and back.

Trans and intersex men are no safer just because they often pass as men. Not only can men be aggressive to each other, particularly young men carrying out what is called in nature the "rutting behaviour", but they can become violent when they discover other men are not like themselves. Females often set one male against another in competition to make the male prove himself by being violent and demonstrating his dominance to be worthy of her. We are, after all is said and done, aggressive animals at times.

Trans men often find this shocking when they transition to live as male. They discover this attitude is one of the most difficult parts of being a man. Consequently, they often do not disclose their trans status for fear of being attacked. Not everyone has the personality, skills, communication skills or wit that can deflect a potential physical attack, particularly if they are in fear of that happening. In the case of Martinez, we can see that no one came to his aid, which is very common crowd behaviour because people are afraid of injury to themselves by getting involved.

Females can also attack trans and intersex people. Chrissy Lee Polis, a 22-year-old trans woman, was trying to use the women's bathroom at McDonalds, Rosedale, Maryland in 2011 when she was viciously attacked by two teenage girls aged 14 and 18 (Siegel, 2011). She was spat at, kicked and punched repeatedly while being dragged along the floor by her hair, resulting in a concussion. The incident was filmed by members of the staff, with other staff being heard laughing in the background, and the video was later put on the internet; the staff members involved were later fired.

Both girls were charged by the police; however, they were not charged with hate crimes. Polis said she believed it was a hate crime. People who stand by and do not report these incidents are clearly complicit and should be charged with being party to the crime, but that rarely happens. Fortunately, Vicky Thomas, a 55-year-old bystander, intervened to stop the attack for fear it would end in a fatality. The victim was shocked when she found out how young her assailants were because they were so strong and violent. The attack left her fearful to go out in public.

People from SGD groups can frequently be attacked by crowds and mobs. In 2018, Miss Suki, a part-time make-up artist and transgender woman, was attacked by several men with sticks and plastic pipes, in Seremban, a town south of Kuala Lumpur in Malaysia (Rising Concerns in the LGBT Community, 2018). She sustained broken ribs, a ruptured spleen and head injuries. Police arrested eight men suspected of carrying out the attack. Miss Suki explained, "They hit me and stepped on me repeatedly; I couldn't move. I tried to call out for help but couldn't speak."

Violence against these communities in Malaysia is believed to be fuelled by radical Muslim groups. There are also attacks against the gay community. As religious extremists become more familiar with utilising the internet to organise themselves, their rhetoric online against these populations becomes more threatening and violent. Trans community leaders say the violence is dramatically increasing and they are living in fear of who may be attacked next.

In India, Hijras are considered the third gender culturally, and consist of trans and intersex people transitioning from younger male roles; they occupy a precarious social space (Gettleman, 2018). Before the British arrived to colonise India, Hijras were part of society and traditionally officiated at weddings and christenings to give blessings for which they were paid. Unfortunately, the British brought with them homophobia and transphobia and embalmed it into Indian life, even creating laws that pushed the Hijras to the margins of society.

It is hard for Hijras to gain work today, so they frequently take to begging or sex work. While they are legally recognised in some parts of India and may even receive a state pension, it is very hard for them to be accepted in mainstream society. At times, they have worked as debt collectors to frighten people into paying what they owe. Some have completed college courses but then been unable to get jobs due to prejudice. Others have some teaching work, but generally they are considered lower caste and undesirable.

In Pakistan, Nayyab Ali was one of four trans women who

stood for parliament in 2018 (Zulfiqar & Victoria, 2018). While trans people have held parliamentary positions in other places, Pakistan is a deeply conservative country. The khawaja sira, Pakistan's equivalent to India's Hijras, are still shunned and ridiculed and have difficulties accessing services such as education, work and healthcare. They are once again among the bottom of the social pile.

Ali stands out because she was the victim of an acid attack by an ex-boyfriend that led to extensive facial scarring. This kind of physical attack is commonly suffered by the average woman in this part of the world. Nayyab explains, "Transgender people are being murdered now. There used to be incidents of beating and acid attacks and we were spared, but these days they just kill us."

Local activists, according to Zulfiqar & Victoria, report that almost 60 transgender women had been killed between 2015–2018 in the highly conservative North-Western province of Khyber Pakhtunkhwa. Another trans woman standing at the elections, Maria Khan, said, "Our own family hires people to murder us. I barely survived an assassination attempt when shots were fired at my house in Mansehra. There are still bullet holes all over my front door."

In the documentary *Middle Sexes* (Thomas, 2005), Calpernia Adams summed up the physical attacks on trans people by saying, "The violence against our community of transgender women seems to be really just over the top, angry and horrible. Usually a transgender woman is not just punched or beaten up or just murdered with gunshot. There are transgender women who are shot with machine guns until they are just pieces of meat, until they are unrecognisable. There are women who are stabbed 30, 40, 50 times and then set on fire. If you could just imagine the time it would take to stab someone 40 times."

Adams also talked about how her boyfriend, who was a solider, knew she was a transsexual woman and they had a loving relationship. However, when his fellow soldiers learned he was dating a trans woman, they used a baseball bat to beat him to death. So the insults, violence and social persecution reaches far beyond the individual themselves.

In 2018, a 36-year-old trans woman, Kelly Stough, from Detroit City's Palmer Park neighbourhood, was shot dead (Fitzsimons, 2018). Albert Weathers, a 46-year-old preacher was charged by the Wayne County prosecutor's office with her murder. Reportedly, Weathers called the police to report an attempted robbery, giving that as the reason he had shot Stough. The police, however, did not believe Weathers and indicated they believe the murder was motivated by Stough's trans status. Under the Trump administration, violent crimes against people from SGD groups rose as his own transphobia infected the nation's radicals.

In an interview with NBC Stough's mother said, "She has a family who cared about her, who loved her, and I want them to know that transgender ladies, expressly those of color, they're just not throwaways; people care about them. She was educated, she was God-filled, she loved church, she loved others. As a human being in the United States of America, you have the right to be who you want to be, and you shouldn't be shamed or bullied or persecuted for the choice you make."

In Argentina, Gabriel David Marino was handed a life sentence for the murder of Diana Sacayán, a well-known trans rights activist (Duffy, 2018b). It was deemed a hate crime as he and his unidentified co-murderer were said to have killed her on the basis of her trans status. Sacayán was violently stabbed to death in her home near Buenos Aires in 2015. At 39, she was renowned as a long-term public trans activist and was the first trans woman to have her gender status recognised in the country.

In South America, a prosecution like this was a triumph, but such cases are generally brought and driven forward by family and community pressure rather than the legal system itself. Many people who come from SGD groups, however, have been excommunicated and shunned by their birth families, are unable to have children, suffer social rejection and live a lot of their lives in isolated loneliness. There is no one to fight for their rights when they are bullied, harassed, experience violence or are murdered.

Intersex murders are poorly recorded as an entity in themselves as most intersex people pass in society as male or female, unnoticed by the general population, so they do not attract so much attention. Many trans and androgynous people are also intersex, so it is impossible to differentiate those intersex people who are a sub-category of the trans population. What we do know is that when people present themselves as intersex in public, they run the same risks of social exclusion and attack that trans populations do because they are outside the stereotypical norm.

The rate of violence that intersex, trans and all SGD groups of people experience is high. There are relentless hate crimes, fuelled by prejudice and discrimination. When you are recognised or known publicly to be from SGD groups, you are othered and recognised as being from a minority. You become vulnerable to bullies, angry people and paranoid groups looking for enemies. They bring with them accumulated aggression and violence that needs a place to land.

Most recorded murders and attacks upon intersex and trans people are perpetrated by males against people identifying as trans females. Males are naturally more aggressive due to higher testosterone levels and high risk-taking behaviours in younger males. These crimes are generally committed by people with lower levels of education, a history of aggressive behaviour, low levels of self-control and fear of being seen as gay. As such, not only are these attacks driven by transphobia but also homophobia. The perpetrators may have had no contact with people from SGD groups before, and so have not developed empathy towards them. They may have been taught that such people are inherently wrong and out to trick them into having improper relations with them. Such attacks are more prevalent where general violent crime rates are higher.

Haaretz (Murders of Transgender People, 2019) reports there have been over 3,000 identified murders of trans people worldwide over the past decade, with common causes being shooting, stabbing and beating, and the level of violence is rising. This does not, of course, include unreported cases or cases that cannot be clearly identified as trans attacks, so we are likely facing at least double those figures. Activists recorded 369 cases within the last year, which is one per day, all more than likely being hate crimes. Brazil was the most dangerous place, with 167 murdered in the past year, compared to 71 in Mexico and 28 in the USA. Three quarters of those cases in the USA were against people from ethnic derivation. Media reports can often refer to these victims as their previous registered sex and gender, an act of malicious gross disrespect.

The list of trans people murdered is a horror chamber of human depravity. For the perpetrator, however, it rarely carries with it the gravitas of sentencing and consequences such hate crimes deserve. Many murderers in these cases claim they suffered the sudden shock of finding out a date was trans and that this pushed them into the panic defence. They justify their actions, saying they were not of their right mind when they committed the murder. These murderers, however, are brutal, violent and clearly terrifyingly mindful in their actions.

At the time of writing, some countries still do not recognise trans people's right to exist or change their sex and gender status. Even in countries that do recognise their status, there may not be laws that offer legal protection against sex- and gender-based discrimination and violence. In countries where there is recognition and sex and gender discrimination laws, it still may be hard for people to be protected because public education has not taught ordinary people about the need to provide fair, human treatment to these groups of people. A country's legal responsibility does not always reflect its willingness to engage in social responsibility.

As of 2021, there are only a few countries that recognise people who do not identify themselves as male or female and wish to have or need documentation to reflect their intersex or sex and/or gender-specific variant status. Some countries offer better rights to intersex people to establish identity than people who simply identify other than male or female. Not only does all of this leave these people outside the legal norms at times, but it puts them at odds with the law and demonises them in society's mind, making them vulnerable. It is a violent act of erasure of identity and body fascism.

The United Nations' (UN) conflation of issues associated with being gay, lesbian or bisexual with those of being from a SGD group confuses the public (United Nations, 2019). The "LGBTIQ" spaghetti label does not work for many people from intersex groups nor for many trans groups. Sexuality is not the defining factor in their sex and gender status for most people from SGD groups. Often, the funding for their care ends up controlled by predominately LGB groups and SGD groups miss out on the funds and care.

The UN's actions on protecting the rights of women, gay men, lesbians, bisexuals and SGD groups is currently woefully inadequate. It promotes its so-called "historic resolution" on protecting people on the grounds of sexual orientation and gender identity but does little in practice (Human Rights Watch, 2019). Many member states not only completely ignore the rights of these people, but they also persecute and legally condone their murder. The UN does not seek sanctions against states for their actions or inactions on these issues, thereby being complicit in those crimes against humanity.

Simply making statements and recommendations about equal rights does not make it so, and if it were other groups in the world receiving such treatment, the UN's members would seek a resolution to take action.

Meanwhile, the World Health Organization (WHO) makes inaccurate and unsubstantiated scaremongering statements such as, "Transgender women are around 49 times more likely to be living with HIV than other adults of reproductive age with an estimated worldwide HIV prevalence of 19%" (WHO, 2019). This is clearly untrue as the populations studied in this research are biased towards sex workers due to where data collection for the projects is carried out. Many trans women are not and have never been sex workers. They access private medical care and therefore do not come in contact with these projects at the same rate as sex workers.

Trans men tend to have less exposure to HIV than the heteronormative population, and many people who now identify under the label "transgender" have low or no sexual encounters and have never used needles. Such bad research and reckless public statements puts fear into the public's mind about people from SGD groups.

The constant confusion between being trans and intersex is common as sex education is not properly being taught in school. Consequently, those who are transphobic also attack intersex people. For the large part, intersex people remain unseen by the public for fear of persecution, violence and attacks. They spend much of their lives in the shadows, unknown to the public, sometimes spending their whole lives trying to deal with unnecessary surgeries or procedures forced upon them as children in order to assimilate them into heteronormality.

This is the backdrop that sets the scene for many people's expectations of being from a SGD group. It can be a grim reality when you are seeing it from a place of disadvantage and your prospects both short- and long-term can seem frightening.

Many people from SGD groups have not been exposed to strong and resilient intersex, trans and other SGD role models, so they can feel isolated, full of self-doubt, depressed and fearful, which leads to suicidation.

The trauma is also intergenerational and has been happening for over 150 years since the acceleration of the medical, over-pathological classification of SGD groups of people. The onset of Victorian puritanising and colonising powers sought to wipe out all signs of being other than stereotypically male or female. Intersex people sometimes ended up as sideshows in the circus and medical curiosities, and trans people were relegated to manuals of sexual perversity.

Hopefully, children from SGD groups are shielded from this reality but still much of other people's negative and hostile attitudes towards them can seep through to their unconscious minds. Dealing with their own issues of being intersex, trans, androgynous, non-binary or neuter is significant enough, and we cannot guard them against outside forces all the time, so having to negotiate an often hostile world can tip them over to suicide.

Adults from SGD groups bring with them their difficulties in negotiating their sex or gender status, historical experiences, knowledge of cultural violence and experiences of prejudice, fear, disappointments and anticipation of danger. Not all of us are battle-hardened, and even those of us who are become overwhelmed with minority stress at times. It can be exhausting always having to be on your guard, concerned that you could be attacked in some way. Sometimes that exhaustion makes suicide look like the better and easier way to go.

Even when we flee from danger to what is often perceived as a safer environment, we can run into the arms of abusers. An autopsy was released of a trans woman, 33-year-old Roxsana Hernández Rodriguez, who died in the custody of US Immigration and Customs Enforcement (ICE) (Gillespie, 2018).

She travelled from Honduras and died around nine days after she was transferred to a US immigration facility in New Mexico run by Core Civic. While she suffered from a history of untreated HIV-related issues, when she died, she was extremely dehydrated and a private autopsy found evidence of violent attack, handcuff restraints trauma and blunt force trauma. Beatings and rape of trans women in prison is a common practice, particularly when they are put into male prison populations.

This is a small bird's eye view of the world in which many people from SGD groups live. When helping people from SGD diverse groups to deal with suicide, ask yourself: How was it to walk a mile in our shoes?

SGD people are not a statistic, aberration, disease, perversion, mental illness, mistake, inconvenience or category but simply human beings who are constantly exposed to minority stress that can drive us at times to thoughts of suicide.

References

Berkovic, N. (2019, February 6). Trans pressing their case. *The Australian*.

Collison, C. (2018, January 24). Intersex babies killed at birth because 'they're bad omens'. *Mail & Guardian*. Retrieved from https://mg.co.za/article/2018-01-24-00-intersex-babies-killed-at-birth-because-theyre-bad-omens

Duffy, N. (2018a, April 16). Piers Morgan claims gender-fluid people are 'damaging to society'. *PinkNews*. Retrieved from https://www.pinknews.co.uk/2018/04/16/piers-morgan-claims-genderfluid-people-are-damaging-to-society/

Duffy, N. (2018b, June 19). Man who murdered Argentina transgender activist Diana Sacayán jailed for life on hate crime charge. *PinkNews*. Retrieved from https://www.pinknews.co.uk/2018/06/19/diana-sacayan-transgender-murder-hate-crime-charge-life-sentence/

Farquhar, G. (2009, August 21). Semenya's sex test explained. *BBC*. Retrieved from http://www.bbc.co.uk/blogs/gordonfarquhar/2009/08/this_must_be_an_awful.html

Fitzsimons, T. (2018, December 13). Detroit pastor charged with transgender woman's murder. *NBC*. Retrieved from https://www.nbcnews.com/feature/nbc-out/detroit-pastor-charged-transgender-woman-s-murder-n947236

Gettleman, J. (2018, February 17). The peculiar position of India's third gender. *New York Times*. Retrieved from https://www.nytimes.com/2018/02/17/style/india-third-gender-hijras-transgender.html

Gillespie. (2018). Trans woman probably physically abused in ICE custody before death, report says. *Fortune*. Retrieved from http://fortune.com/2018/11/26/trans-woman-probably-physically-abused-in-ice-custody-before-death-report-says

Hitler, A. (1992). *Mein Kampf.* Vintage.

Human Rights Watch. (2016, June 30). UN makes history on sexual orientation, gender identity. Retrieved from https://www.hrw.org/news/2016/06/30/un-makes-history-sexual-orientation-gender-identity

Jackman, J. (2017, May 17). Piers Morgan calls non-binary children 'a contagion' as he attacks trans couple. *PinkNews*. Retrieved from https://www.pinknews.co.uk/2018/04/16/piers-morgan-claims-genderfluid-people-are-damaging-to-society/

Jacks, T. (2019, February 4). 'I take a risk when I get on': Transgender commuters describe life on public transport. *The Age*. Retrieved from www.theage.com.au/national/victoria/i-take-a-risk-when-i-get-on-transgender-commuters-describe-life-on-public-transport-20190201-p50v1x.html

Martínez-Patiño, M. J. (2005). Personal Account: A woman tried and tested. *Lancet*. 366: S38. Retrieved from https://www.thelancet.com/pdfs/journals/lancet/PIIS0140673605678415.pdf

Murders of transgender people rising worldwide (2019, February 7). *Haaretz*. Retrieved from www.haaretz.com/world-news/murders-of-transgender-people-rising-worldwide-1.6674858

Paris transgender woman 'humiliated' at protest. (2019, April 3). *BBC News*. Retrieved from https://www.bbc.com/news/world-europe-47799288

Rising concerns in the LGBT community after attack on transgender women. (2018, August 4). *The Straits Times*. Retrieved from https://www.straitstimes.com/asia/se-asia/a-brutal-assault-and-rising-fear-in-malaysias-lgbt-community

Siegel, A. (2011, August 4). Teen pleads guilty to beating transgender woman at Rosedale McDonald's. *The Baltimore Sun*. Retrieved from https://www.baltimoresun.com/news/maryland/baltimore-county/bs-md-co-mcdonalds-beating-plea-20110804-story.htm

Sosin, K. (2018, December 14). Trans man in Pittsburgh beaten in alleged hate crime. Retrieved from https://www.intomore.com/impact/trans-man-in-pittsburgh-beaten-in-alleged-hate-crime

Stark, J. (2017, May 9). For some transgender students, the school bathroom is a battleground. Retrieved from www.abc.net.au/news/2017-04-01/transgender-students-bathroom-battleground/8395782

The Williams Institute, UCLA School of Law (2017, January 17). New estimates show that 150,000 youth ages 13 to 17 identify as transgender in the US. Retrieved from https://williamsinstitute.law.ucla.edu/research/transgender-issues/new-estimates-show-that-150000-youth-ages-13-to-17-identify-as-transgender-in-the-us/

Thomas, A. [TyneTrans]. 2005. Middle sexes—redefining he and she. Retrieved from https://www.youtube.com/watch?v=Gyoq6tdlsE

United Nations. (2019, February). LGBT people have been part of all societies throughout history. Retrieved from https://www.unfe.org/sexual-orientation-gender-identity-nothing-new

Visentin, L. (2015, December 1). Man who bashed transgender woman at Newtown pub given community service. *Sydney Morning Herald*. Retrieved from https://www.smh.com.au/national/nsw/man-who-bashed-transgender-woman-at-newtown-pub-given-community-service-20151201-glclow.html

World Health Organization. (2019). Transgender people. Retrieved from https://www.who.int/hiv/topics/transgender/about/en/

Zulfiqar, A., & Victoria, B. (2018, July). The transgender acid attack survivor running for parliament. *BBC News*. Retrieved from https://www.bbc.com/news/world-asia-44684714

Chapter 2:
Who Are Sex Diverse People?

Sex and/or gender diverse (SGD) groups of people have existed for as long as biological life has emerged on the planet and subdivided, evolving from simple self-reproducing organisms like archaea, bacteria and some self-reproducing plants, to multi-sex species that require the fusion of gametes. Self-reproducing single-sex organisms generally have the same chromosomes and genes as their parent cell; but when two or more sexes are needed to reproduce, it becomes a genetic game of "shake the snow globe" to see how the chromosomes will land. In comparison to humans, for example, the Schizophyllum Commune fungi have 23,328 distinct mating types.

Again, I remind you, the reader, this chapter is not a medical text but seeks to give you some background information on some of the physical ways your clients will present. Having a background knowledge will aid you in building rapport with the client.

Humans, like many other, but obviously not all, forms of life have two basic sexes of male and female. Around 20 years ago, I calculated and estimated a 1% to 2% variant of the population are born with, sometimes pronounced and sometimes not, developmental amorphous sex anomalies and gender diversity. These can be obvious at birth or not depending on the individual. Some children become intersex not because of genetic anomalies but due to growth differences in the womb, leading to congenital birth defects, organ failure, hypotrophy, hypertrophy, hypoactivity or hyperactivity.

Sex is made up of many factors:

1. Birth attendant determination on observation of gonads, how the genitals appear to others and what sex you were registered as at birth (natal sex).
2. Body characteristics (phenotype) of whether you aesthetically appear male or female, both or neither.
3. Developmental growth of ancillary sex features such as vagina, breasts, fallopian tubes, uterus, cervix, penis, epididymis, prostate, ejaculatory ducts and vas deferens.
4. Gonadal presence of ovaries, testes, ovotestes or their absence, function or dysfunction.
5. Brain determination and development, pituitary gland function, volume of corpus callosum, typical or atypical brain anatomy.
6. Circulating hormonal levels of oestrogens, progesterone and androgens from your gonads, adrenal glands, adipose tissue, oestrogen biosynthesis by aromatase activity in the brain, and extra glandular production.
7. The genetics of how many X or Y chromosomes, or partial X and Y, you may or may not have in the whole or various parts of your body, with the usual male having 46 XY chromosomes and females having 46 XX. They not only determine tissue formation but also how enzymes hormones and other body biochemicals behave.
8. Psychological sex determines how your cognitive functions, behaviours and emotional patterns manifest and how you perceive yourself.
9. Self-perceived sex fantasy of how you psychologically construct your sex interactions with self and others in relationship to your body.
10. Your spiritual sense of your sex, which is individual to you, as in many cultures physical sex is intrinsically linked to spirituality.

11. Social sex around how you act out your own body in family, social or work groups and society in general.
12. Historical sex in how long you have been recognised as one sex or another and what history goes with that identification.
13. Cosmetic sex in how you are constructing your sex through alteration of its appearance through hormones or surgery.
14. Legal sex status in society of whether you are considered male, female, intersex or sex non-specific, which gives you legal access to social spaces, privileges and protection.

I am now going to revise my previous sex and gender variance figure to well over 1–2% of the human population. The reasons why, as we shall see, is that genetics has greatly advanced since I last published on this more than two decades ago (O'Keefe, 1999). We can now track cell lines to find the existence of simultaneous XX and XY cell lines in many of the populations (chimeras) So being intersex, sex diverse or sex different is no longer as marginal, obvious or initially medically detectable. In most cases, it does not present as a medical emergency and its effects are on a gradient scale from undetectable to physiological dysfunction. Not only does intersex include aneuploidy (non-average number of chromosomes) but also huge physiological variations. So, the occurrences of intersex and sex variance is now much more widely observed.

Being intersex or sex variant, however, does not always begin before birth but is also the result of development occurrences, environmental influences, disease, trauma, iatrogenic drug use and medical procedures and treatments throughout life that can have nothing at all to do with genetics as the origin. It can begin to happen at any age and renders the person in the area between stereotypically male and female. Some of the causes of this we know about, and some science is only just beginning to discover as we map the human and other species' biological experience.

When you explore and work in the area of suicide prevention in SGD groups of people, you need to understand about the biological as well as psychological experiences of your clients. Anything else is like trying to drive a taxi through the streets of New York with a blindfold on.

I delicately play a game of diplomacy in this text between the word 'condition' (noting medical dysfunction) and 'occurrence'. A condition is when there is a medical problem, as with some intersex conditions. For many intersex people, who have no medical emergency, they consider that the occurrence of their intersex status is a variance in nature and not a deformation, disease or condition that needs medical intervention. They can become offended when described as having a condition or being seen as wrong and abnormal. However, I am sometimes going to refer to those occurrences as conditions from a medical point of view because they do cause medical problems.

For these reasons, I use the phrase 'sex diverse', not to rob other intersex people of their identity as intersex, but simply to emphasise that we are not only male, female and intersex but a whole host of diversity in our sex presentations. Neither do I seek to rob someone of any disease or condition status that affords them the right to medical treatment.

There is a belief with certain intersex rights campaigners that being intersex means the presence of atypical male or female genitals; however, this is not strictly the case. Anomalies can occur due to genetics, genital differences, reproductivity, endocrinological reasons, nutritional dysfunction, brain differences, trauma consequences, disease, cancers, iatrogenic alteration, radiation, chemotherapy, toxic disrupters, and hormonal imbalance in the mother's or parent's womb.

Common Physical Variants

Gynecomastia is a hormone disorder that results in males growing excessive breast tissue (Johnson & Murad, 2009). It can be the results of genetic variance, metabolic dysfunction, decline in testosterone, diseases, certain cancers, medication side effects, obesity, dietary or toxic poisoning, and occur anytime of life. Treatment may require aromatase inhibitors or surgical or liposuction removal of the unwanted breast tissue. It does not necessarily preclude fertility but can be associated with infertile conditions.

Male Hypogonadism results in small testes, low androgen output or insensitivity and failure to masculinise, including at times infertility. Primarily present at birth or secondly as a developmental failure during growth. The causes are genetic defects, hypopituitarism, Kallmann Syndrome, Klinefelter Syndrome, Kartagener Syndrome, Androgyne Insensitivity Syndrome, trauma, brain damage, tumours, disease, anorexia, malnutrition, toxic hormone interrupters, birth parent's use of opioids inducing androgen deficiency with drugs such as codeine, dihydrocodeine, morphine, oxycodone, methadone, fentanyl, hydromorphone, endocrine disruptor diethylstilbestrol, anabolic steroid-induced hypogonadism in males, childhood mumps, high levels of oestrogen in the womb, ageing testicular atrophy, radiotherapy and chemotherapy. In some cases, testosterone treatment can increase fertility (Thirumalai et al., 2017).

Female Hypogonadism resulting in absent, small, low or non-functioning ovaries, which are the result of brain damage, congenital adrenal hyperplasia, complete Androgyne Insensitivity Syndrome where hidden testes are present, Turner's syndrome, hypopituitarism, low human growth hormone, metabolic disruption, toxic hormone disrupters, disease, anorexia, malnutrition, medication-induced hormone disruption, radiation, chemotherapy (Richard-Eaglin, 2018). In some cases, fertility can be restored with oestrogen and progesterone treatment.

Hypospadias & Chordee occurs when urination voids from the underside of the penis (hypospadias) not its tip and the penis is bent forward (chordee). It affects around one in every 250 to 300 male births and needs surgical correction for normal urination and sexual intercourse later in life (van der Horst & de Wall, 2017). Controversially, this is often left out of intersex conditions, but it may be due to hormonal failure to develop, so it is intersex-related.

Cryptorchidism is the failure of one of more testicles to descend down the inguinal canal into the scrotum. It occurs in about 3% of all full-term male births, 30% of premature births and can result in testicular failure and reduced fertility. Most testes descend in the first month or years but the longer they remain undescended the greater the likelihood of hypogonadism, increased testicular germ cell tumours, torsion, inguinal hernias, psychological problems and even testicular failure (Varela-Cives et al., 2015).

Ovotestes are a gonadal mixture of ovarian and testicular tissue. Originally, all gonads start by developing from the bipotential gonad (a "streak" of cells called the genital ridge) in XY embryos at about 12 weeks after conception when SRY-SOX9 kicks in. DMRT1, a protein produced by the DMRT1 gene, stabilises testes (in its absence, ovaries develop).

Gonadal damage due to trauma, polytrauma and disease occurs, leading to gonadal functional failure (Faucher et al., 2010). Males and females can lose their gonads to accidents, disease or cancer where an orchidectomy is needed. Gonads are also rendered dysfunctional due to mumps in males, radiation treatment and chemotherapy. In children, this can lead to failure to develop at puberty and in adults, it may lead to partial virilisation in females and demasculinisation in males. Hormone replacement therapy is not always possible, particularly if the patient has liver issues or cardiovascular disease, rendering such treatment contraindicated. Fertility is compromised along with a reduction and failure in the primary and secondary sex characteristics and functions.

Menopause and ADAM (Androgen Decline in Aging Males) not only leads to reduced levels of androgens, oestrogens, progesterone but also causes aging-related hypogonadism. In males as androgens reduce, if excess weight is gained, then adipose tissues increase oestrogen effects, which can lead to physiological emasculation and feminising effects. In females, the reduction in oestrogen and progesterone can cause adrenal androgens to seem more potent, reducing breast size, deepening of the voice and producing facial hair in some females. These hormonal changes can affect structures within the aging brain (Zárate et al., 2017). Also, some adrenal androgens like DHEA can be reduced with aging, which reduces energy and potential of aggressiveness, although in cases of senile dementia, Alzheimer's and mental illness that may not be the case.

These causative conditions below will contribute to physical variants:

Congenital Adrenal Hyperplasia (CAH) are several autosomal recessive conditions resulting in gene mutations in the CYP21A gene for enzymes which mediate biochemical production of mineralocorticoids, glucocorticoids or sex steroids from cholesterol by the adrenal glands (Steroidogenesis is the process when cholesterol is converted to biologically active steroid hormones). A lot of these conditions invoke deficient or excessive production of sex hormones that can lead to a child's and adult's primary and secondary sex characteristics being altered. The various forms of CAH are associated with producing symptoms such as vomiting due to salt wasting, ambiguous genitalia, early pubic hair and rapid growth in childhood, precocious puberty, delayed puberty, under and over viralisation, menstrual irregularities, excessive facial hair, enlarged clitoris, shallow vagina, hypogonadism and infertility. Medication and hospitalisation may be required, for life in some cases. A percentage of children can be prone to regular hospitalisation (Yang & White, 2017).

Non-classic Congenital Adrenal Hyperplasia Due to 21-hydroxylase Deficiency (NCAH) can produce excess virilisation at puberty and can give rise to classic cases of late onset intersex physiological changes in females. While some cases remain undetected with no obvious symptoms, sudden onset can occur at any age (Witchel & Azziz, 2010).

Complete Androgen Insensitivity Syndrome (CAIS) Reifenstein Syndrome), androgen deficiency syndromes are due to an X-linked recessive androgen receptor defect in 46, XY children. They can be born with a vagina, clitoris, no ovaries or womb, or partial female genital development, internal testes and have XY chromosomes. However, without androgen receptors on the surface of the cell, androgens can have no expression so secondary sex characteristics, including genitalia, develop as female. Occurrence is around one in every 13,000 births and they are infertile (Lanciotti et al., 2019).

Partial Androgen Insensitivity Syndrome (PAIS) androgen deficiency syndromes are due to partial ability for androgen hormone binding. The androgens are only partly metabolised.

This leads to children developing genitals on a gradient on the male scale with testes, but still partly insensitive to androgens. The male genitalia is partially or not fully masculinised. Occurrence is rare with infertility present and often going undiagnosed, creating difficulty in clinical classification (Lucas-Herald et al., 2016).

Mild Androgen Insensitivity Syndrome (MAIS) androgen deficiency syndromes are due to greater ability for androgen hormone binding but not sufficient for full typical male development. Here the child is mildly insensitive to androgens but normal male external genitalia is formed. The insensitivity is enough to impair spermatogenesis. The individual is infertile and may be hypogonadal. Research is sparse in this area although in a few cases greater virilisation has been achieved for some time now in some patients with androgen supplementation (Weidemann et al., 1998).

Klinefelter Syndrome (KS) (also known as 47,XXY or XXY) is where there are two or more X chromosomes plus a Y, resulting in small testes and infertility. It is sometimes recognised as the most common genetically-caused intersex disorder, occurring in around two in 1,000 births. Boys can grow taller than other boys, have incomplete genital and gonadal development, a micropenis, reduced sex drive, gynecomastia, propensity to put on weight around the girth, weaker muscles, retarded motor development, reduced facial and body hair, cognitive impairment, memory loss, problems with speech, dyslexia and depression (Nieschlag et al., 2016). Treatment with testosterone can increase function and masculinisation. Fertility has been recorded in some cases due to the use of IVF techniques with extracted sperm.

XXYY Syndrome Karyotype, a variant of Klinefelter's syndrome, occurs with the inclusion of an extra X and Y chromosome, leading to developmental and functional problems, which can include hypogonadism, learning difficulties, cognitive processing difficulties, intellectual challenges, mood disorders, seizures, elbow malformations and concerns with bone and muscles strength, often treated with testosterone (Tartaglia et al., 2011). Fertility has been assisted through IVF treatment in some cases (De-Feng et al., 2018).

45,X/46,XY Mosaicism (X0/XY Mosaicism, Mixed Gonadal Dysgenesis) is a variation of sex chromosome aneuploidy and mosaicism of the Y chromosome. It gives rise to partial virilisation, ambiguous genitalia and even complete male and female reproductive systems. Müllerian ducts and Wolffian ducts may be asymmetrical with a high risk of gonadoblastoma (tumour). Variation can range from gonadal dysgenesis (functionless fibrous tissues) in males to Turner's-like symptoms in females, and short stature. Persons can experience infertility (Akinsal et al., 2018).

Human Male/Female Chimeras are individuals who have two sets of DNA, one male and one female. They may be fertile females who have absorbed a male twin's DNA during gestation and now have a line of XY cells growing in their body, a mother who has absorbed the DNA of a male child during pregnancy or the results of a bone marrow transplant. They may also be males who have absorbed a female twin's DNA during twin death invitro, known as vanishing twin syndrome. They are not hybrids but naturally occurring chimeras, and it is posited that up to 1 in 30 of births originally start as multiple births, with 20% loss during gestation. If this happens during IVF treatment, an adverse pregnancy outcome can occur (Zhou et al., 2016). It is even posited that different systems in the body may have different DNA, with one being typically male or female. It can lead to variations of sex development during pregnancy. Some women who are chimera are fertile.

Freemartin Syndrome is the result of a female child being masculinised by her male twin's blood hormone levels and absorbing some of his DNA, a form of chimerism. This can lead to failure of female reproductive development. While common in cattle, it has been cited to exist in humans (Bogdanova et al., 2010).

Swyer Syndrome (46,XY complete gonadal dysgenesis) individuals have an X chromosome and Y chromosome in each cell, the pattern typically found in what can be presumed to be boys and men but may present as female. They can have female reproductive structures and external genitalia that can present as ambiguous. This is due to mutations of the SRY gene. Occurrence is around one in every 80,000 births. Gonadal dysgenesis (conditions that can cause impaired development of the gonads) is present that can become cancerous and is usually removed. Hormone replacement therapy can be used at times to induce menstruation and produce female secondary sex characteristics, breast enlargement and womb development, helping reduce osteopenia and osteoporosis. Pregnancy and successful birth by C-section at 39 weeks has been recorded by IVF with a donation egg therapy (Taneja et al., 2016).

Turner's Syndrome (Monosomy X, 45X and Ullrich-Turner Syndrome) is a genetic condition that affects women who only have one X chromosome instead of two. Generally involving 20% of conceptus, 99% die or abort before birth. The individual may present with short stature, infertility, congenital heart disease, hypertension, kidney structural problems, thyroid dysregulation, type II diabetes, spatial awareness issues, absence of menstruation, vision and hearing problems, sunken wide chest, with broadly spaced nipples, webbed skin on neck, puffy hands, elbow extension issues, soft upturned nails, and low hairline. This condition affects around one in every 2,000 women.

Research using magnetic resonance imaging shows structural brain differences in girls with Turner's that account for cognitive processing difficulties (Hong & Reiss, 2012).

XYY Syndrome is where a male has an extra Y chromosome. Boys can grow taller than average and childhood acne can occur. It is not an inherited condition but the results of a random deviation in sperm formation that occurs in around one in every 1,000 fathers. Neither is it classically an intersex condition but simply a chromosome anomaly with fertility remaining normal but we list it as a sex variance (Aksglaede et al., 2008).

XXX Syndrome (Trisomy X) is the most common variance in females, occurring in about one in 1,000 female births, largely undetected, again not being a classically intersex condition but a chromosome anomaly. A range of variations occur including seizures, renal, gastrointestinal and genitourinary variations, and early ovarian failure, tall stature, epicanthal folds, hypotonia and clinodactyly (Tartaglia et al., 2010).

5-Alpha Reductase Deficiency is an intersex recessive autosome condition that affects male sexual development before birth and during puberty in one in every 4,500 births. There is lack of 5-alpha reductse which is the enzyme that converts testosterone into dihydrotestosterone responsible for male development. Persons are genetically male with one X and Y chromosome in each cell and formed testes, but until puberty, they generally can be mistaken as female due to an underdeveloped penis and undescended testes. At adolescence when a testosterone hormone surge occurs, underdeveloped tissue develops into a small penis. So initially the person may be brought up as female, with some deciding to live as male later and occasionally some deciding to live as female (Nascimento et al., 2018).

Transexed, Transsexual and Transgender are all labels that are used by people who do not identify as their registered natal sex, with many seeking to change their bodies through hormones and surgery to reflect a different sex, whether that be male, female or neuter. Kruijver et al. (2000) found male to female transsexuals had female neuron numbers in the limbic nucleus in the brain. Bakker (2018) reported a study using magnetic resonance that scanned brain differences in children and adolescents complaining of sex and gender dysphoria; their brains were more akin to the brains of their desired sex. Also, gene expression may be deviating hormonal activation from its usual course.

This confirms findings found in Holland back in the 1990s and 2000s, suggesting that at times where the genital development is going in one direction the brain may be developing in another, due to hormonal disruption or failure or genetic differences (Kruijver et al., 2000). There is now clear scientific evidence to include many of these people in the intersex group since many are sex variant.

Mayer-Rokitansky-Kuster-Hauser (MRKH) Syndrome (Mullerian Aplasia) is vaginal agenesis when the vagina does not develop during gestation, leading to a partial blind pouch with a roof or the complete absence of a vagina, plus a failure of uterine development and absence of the cervix, occurring in one in every 4,500 to 5,000 females. In some cases, external genitalia may appear normal. There can be normally functioning ovaries. Type 1 is genital malformation only while type 2 can give rise to ear, skeletal, heart and kidney problems. Management usually requires surgery to create a vagina (Herlin et al., 2020); and some successful experiments with hormone administration have resulted in maturation of the uterus. Egg generation can be possible through IVF, allowing pregnancy (Raziel et al., 2012).

Acromegaly occurs in the presence of excess human growth hormone (HGH) produced by the pituitary gland, so the person grows excessively. This condition is often referred to as gigantism, where the person displays enlarged hands, feet, forehead, nose, jaw, deepening of the voice, joint problems, thickening of the skin, headaches, vision problems, high blood pressure, sleep apnoea, type II diabetes, heart failure, kidney failure, colorectal cancer, arthritis, and carpel tunnel syndrome. According to the National Institute of Diabetes and Digestive and Kidney Diseases ("National Institute of Diabetes and Digestive and Kidney Disease," n.d.), acromegaly affects three to 14 in every 100,000 people. This produces an overly-masculinised appearance in both in males and females. In 95% of cases, this overproduction is due to a pituitary tumour and surgery can be attempted to remove that tissue. Sometimes it is due to tumours in other parts of the body. Radiation and drug therapy are used to slow HGH production (Lenders et al., 2020).

Cloacal Exstrophy is where there are birth defects of the entire pelvic region that can cause the reproductive system, intestines and bladder to be deformed due to poor development of the ventral body wall. There can be an absence or malformation of the genital and reproductive system. It is sometimes argued that this is not an intersex condition, but many males have been reassigned as females after emergency surgery. These decisions were made by medical staff because they believed there was insufficient genital tissue to support a male identity (Reiner & Gearhart, 2002). However, there is reporting that shows a high level of patient dissatisfaction with this decision. Because this is sex-variant, we treat this as an intersex condition.

Sex Determining Genetics
Many people who experience sex diversity have rare genetic variants that contribute towards the outcome of their physiology.

Here it is not possible to discuss all of them. The discovery of the SRY gene in the 1990s was a major sex development turning point in genetics as various mutations cause varying degrees of genetic failures and produce rare reproductive system development differences (Hawkins et al., 1992).

There are, of course, other variants that cause sex differences. Each of the several forms of CAH are associated with a specific sex chromosome aneuploidy (Grošelj et al., 2016). In Down Syndrome, a variant also affects sex development and most of the time causes infertility (Stefanidis et al., 2011); variants in the SRD5A2 gene causes deficiency of alpha reductase that affects supply of male hormone when male children first appear female then undergo penile growth at puberty (Hiort et al., 2002). In the case of Klinefelter's and XYY Syndrome, people can have an extra chromosome that affects development.

A study (Foreman et al., 2019) found a significant association between sex and gender dysphoria and ERα, SRD5A2, and STS alleles, as well as ERα and SULT2A1 genotypes. The study involved 390 transgender women who had transitioned or were in the process of doing so. However, the label 'transgender' strays into a grey area of being a limited description that does not always encompass some people who transition, corrupting the participant pools. It does show us, however, that sex differentiation genetically goes far beyond what may be presently assessed medically. It also opens up the wide realisation that so many of us as humans are sex variant, just as we have different hair or eye colour.

We must also consider that it is not always just one genetic variant, failure or absence that affects sex development and function. It can also be a combination of differing genes, their interaction, sometimes at idiosyncratic levels, and enzyme failures that lead to unusual sex differences.

So how do we get to 2%-plus of the population being sex variant?

Well, we start by adding up all of the people who are identified as intersex, sex diverse, sex affected and altered by age and environment, those who have genetic anomalies that deviate from the stereotypical 46 XX or XY male/female chromosome format. Then we include the average 10% of the population who are infertile due to reproductive failure for any reason which renders them other than fully reproductive males or females. At this point, we probably go into double figures percentage-wise for sex diversity. Just because you cannot see it with the naked eye, and we cannot presently detect it, does not mean it is not occurring.

Fertility

Many intersex and sex diverse people experience infertility. For some people from intersex and sex diverse groups, at the moment, there is no knowledge available that allows them the option of fertility. For some, fertility may happen naturally and for others, it may be induced. There are also those who may have bodies that would not physically support fertilsation, gestation and birth.

We are considering these issues because infertility can lead to depression, in many cases increasing the risks of suicide. Since many SGD groups of people suffer profound familial and social rejection, plus infertility, they often end up not connected to families or communities and can live in isolation, sometimes developing attachment problems. They may still experience the yearning for a family, leading to a high level of anxiety and depression. I have previously referred to this as Chronic Childlessness Syndrome.

Let us first define what we are talking about when we are discussing fertility. It should be made clear that fertility is primarily the ability to pass on your own genetic material to the next generation, resulting in a live birth. We may include assisted reproductive procedures. This can be achieved by many means and those means will increase in the future.

Increased fertility for those with female reproductive systems may be achieved in some cases, where normal female gonads are present, with administration of follicle-stimulating hormone (FSH), luteinizing hormone (LH) and a range of treatments, provided ancillary reproductive organs are present. In some cases, this may or may not need IVF intervention.

As we saw earlier (Taneja et al., 2016) induced pregnancy and live birth was achieved in women who experience Swyer Syndrome. During virilisation, due to Polycystic Ovary Syndrome (PCOS) that produced dysmenorrhea and possible infertility, with some patients, fertility can be aided with metformin, clomiphene citrate, or metformin with clomiphene citrate, gonadotropins or laparoscopic weight loss surgery and thyroid management (Melo et al., 2016). Here we do consider PCOS as creating a sex variant, temporary or not.

Fertility and production of sperm has been increased in males experiencing hypogonadism and underviralisation by the administration of hCG with or without hMG/FSH (Ho & Tan, 2013), although it is tempting to treat underviralisation with testosterone anti-estrogens and aromatase inhibitors. While this may have been experimented with in secondary hypogonadism it may open up experimentation in primary cases. However, (Lipshultz et al., 2014) warn that testosterone supplementation can damage existing testicular fertility.

For those with genetic variants who experience intersex or sex diversity due to inherited genetics or a chromosomal defects, new gene splicing techniques like CRISPR may offer ways for gene correction during reproduction (Egli et al., 2018). Ma et al. (2017) recently reconfirmed their progress in gene correction in embryos in *Nature*. While these techniques are in their early days, progress in gene editing and nuclear-transfer (gene substitution) will become common practice in time once more ethical guidelines and laws catch up with the science.

Correcting genetic defects, however, does not help people who do not possess reproductive organs that support gestation or necessarily produce an ovum or sperm. While human cloning of corrected cells and surrogacy might be used to create a mature embryo, we are not yet at that scientific stage, although we may be in time. Cloning in humans is very complex, illegal in many countries, and would take billions of dollars of research as most attempts at cloning fail. Yi Zhang, a stem cell biologist at Boston Children's Hospital, has claimed he has produced chemicals that would increase the success rate to 25%, but ethical permission to clone a whole human being may be very hard to attain (Regalado, 2018).

A more viable option may be the creation of sperm or ovum from stem cells that have undergone processes like CRISPR using gene manipulation and nuclear-transfer. Once again, if the person cannot carry a child, using a surrogate or the womb of a partner could give the genetic links that some people may want to their children. As science progresses, we may arrive at a stage where it might be possible for us all to be both fathers and mothers, provided that progress is not halted by moral concerns around eugenics.

In early 2021, two teams of researchers reported that they could make tiny embryonic blastoids from either stem cells or reprogrammed skin cells by growing them in 3D wells. While this was for the purposes of studying early embryonic problems, and they could not legally keep them for longer than 14 days, this truly opens up the possibility of parthenogenesis in humans (Yu et al., 2021). As I predicted nearly 20 years ago, sooner or later, someone will grow a baby in box somewhere.

In cases where a viable pregnancy may not be possible, surrogacy could be used to grow those embryos and carry the child to birth. The problem at the moment, however, is that heteronormative people have assumed cisgender rights above SGD groups of people and surrogacy is often blocked.

Regenerative medicine is a field that will allow gonadal and ancillary sex organs to be grown in a laboratory in the future. The field of tissue regeneration and generation is no longer science fiction but science fact, even though, it is still in its infancy. Muscular, valvular, cardiac, kidney, forearm and skin tissue generation are already the main areas of research in this field, and this will be followed by reproductive organs, as penis structures have already been achieved. Also, organ 3D printing is being experimented with to print organs from the cells of the patient (Zhang et al., 2021). At the moment, stem cells from amniotic fluid and the placenta seem to aid more in neo-organ formation, so tissue banking before or at birth could render more opportunities to future generations.

This will mean that full organs could be grown outside the body on scaffolding including reproductive organs, from your own stem cells, or even creating altered donor stem cells that will not be rejected. This would avoid the major problem of organ transplant rejection that is holding us back in this area. The future may also involve growing organs within the body itself on frame structures and using nanotechnology. Getting solid (complex with many vessels) organs to function and produce ovum or sperm and mature to pregnancy may be a separate challenge but might not be too far a journey with the scientific progress being made.

Experimentation with womb transfers for AIS and trans women may very soon begin. There have been reports of womb transplants from live donors since 2004. In 2016, a woman who suffered Mayer-Rokitansky-Küster-Hauser Syndrome (MRKH), gave birth by C-section after having had a transplanted womb from a 45-year-old deceased donor who had already carried children (Chmel et al., 2019).

There is a significant number of problems facing transplanting into many intersex women and trans women; the pelvic bones can be too narrow, vascular attachment has challenges as natally developed females tend to have more blood supply, which avoids tissue starvation and atrophy. Also, neo natal vaginas constructed from skin grafts and penile inversion have an acid balance that will not support pregnancy (Jones et al. (2019). However, there is no reason why these anatomical issues cannot be overcome with careful consideration. It is anticipated that a vagina transplant from a deceased body will also be necessary at the same time in order to provide the pH value to support the pregnancy. This will require a revision of the way sex affirmation surgery is carried out.

Many trans men, who have not had a hysterectomy, vaginectomy or oophorectomy, are now getting pregnant and having children. A number of trans men are not having phalloplasty (penile construction) via skin flap resection and/or metoidioplasty because of the expense and high failure rates. It was believed for many years that once HRT testosterone was administered pregnancy would no longer be possible during that treatment. Cases, however, have emerged which show that pregnancy is possible while still injecting those medications even though regular menstruation appears to have stopped. In the documentary *Seahorse* (Finlay, 2019), a trans man Freddie is followed during pregnancy while living as a man, even though he had ceased testosterone treatment.

Saving eggs and sperm pre-transition has been done for around 30 years now for post-transition trans people who had a functional reproductive system, allowing them to have a biological connection to children after their transition. This has been very successful in many cases where relationships have proved stable and even in single trans people using IVF or surrogacy. In other cases, traditionally, many sex diverse people have also used adoption and used donated eggs or sperm to create families by surrogacy.

For many people from sex diverse groups who have the drive to be genetically and biologically connected to their offspring, as we can now see, the future of reproduction in sex diverse people looks interesting, not hopeless, not despairing and not impossible. That hope and promise of human connection in people from sex diverse groups will undoubtedly reduce suicidal ideation for many.

References

Akinsal, E., Baydili, N., Bayramov, & Ekmekcioglu, O. (2017). A rare cause of male infertility: 45,X/46,XY Mosaicism. *Urologia Internationalis.* 101(4), 481–485. doi: 10.1159/000484615

Aksglaede, L., Skakkebaek, N.E., & Juul, A. (2008). Abnormal sex chromosome constitution and longitudinal growth: serum levels of insulin-like growth factor (IGF)-I, IGF binding protein-3, luteinizing hormone, and testosterone in 109 males with 47,XXY, 47,XYY, or sex-determining region of the Y chromosome (SRY)-positive 46,XX karyotypes. *The Journal of Clinical Endocrinology & Metabolism.* 93(1),169–176.

Bakker, J. (2018). Brain structure and function in gender dysphoria. *Endocrine Abstracts.* doi: 10.1530/endoabs.56. S30.3

Bogdanova, N., Siebers, U., Kelsch, R., Markoff, A., Ropke, A., Exeler, R., Tsokas, J., & Wieacker, P. (2010). Blood chimerism in a girl with Down syndrome and possible freemartin effect leading to aplasia of the Müllerian derivatives. *Human Reproduction*, 25(5), 1339–1343. Retrieved from https://doi.org/10.1093/humrep/deq048

Chmel, R., Novackova, M., Libor, J., Matecha, J., Pastor, Z., Maluskova, J., Cekal, M., Kristek, J., Olausson, M., & Fronek, J. (2018, August 27). Revaluation and lessons learned from the first 9 cases of a Czech uterus transplantation trial: Four deceased donor and 5 living donor uterus transplantations, *American Journal of Transplantation*. Wiley Online Library. Retrieved from https://onlinelibrary.wiley.com/doi/full/10.1111/ajt.15096

De-Feng, L., Zhao, L., Hong, K., Yang, Y., Zhang, Z., & Jiang, H. (2018). Fertility achieved through in vitro fertilization in a male patient with 48,XXYY syndrome. *Asian Journal of Andrology*. Retrieved from https://www.ncbi.nlm.nih.gov/pmc/articles/PMC5858110/

Egli, D., Zuccaro, M., Kosicki, M., Church, G., Bradley, A., & Jasin, M. (2018). Inter-homologue repair in fertilized human eggs? *Nature*. Retrieved from https://www.nature.com/articles/s41586-018-0379-5

Faucher, L., Ward, M., Burgess, P., Williams, D., Herrforth, C., & Bentz, M. (2010). Threatened fertility and gonadal function after a polytraumatic, life-threatening injury. *Journal of Emergencies, Trauma, and Shock*. 3(2),199–203. doi: 10.4103/0974-2700.62110

Finlay, J. (Director). (2019). *Seahorse* [Motion picture]. United Kingdom: BBC.

Foreman, M., Hare, L., York, K., Balakrishnan, K., Sánchez, F.J., Harte, F., Erasmus, J., Vilain, E., & Harley, V.R. (2019). Genetic link between gender dysphoria and sex hormone signaling. *The Journal of Clinical Endocrinology & Metabolism*. 104(2), 390–396. Retrieved from: https://doi.org/10.1210/jc.2018-01105

Grošelj, U., Žerjav Tanšek, M., Trebušak Podkrajšek, K., Hovnik, T., Battelino, T., & Dolžan, V. (2016). Clinical role of CYP2C19 polymorphisms in patients with congenital adrenal hyperplasia due to 21-hydroxylase deficiency. *Acta Chimica Slovenica*. 63(1),33–37.

Hawkins, J., Taylor, A., Goodfellow, P., Migeon, C., Smith, K., & Berkovitz, G. (1992). Evidence for increased prevalence of SRY mutations in XY females with complete rather than partial gonadal dysgenesis. *The American Journal of Human Genetics.* 51(5), 979–984.

Herlin, M., Petersen, M., & Brännström, M. (2020). Mayer-Rokitansky-Küster-Hauser (MRKH) syndrome: a comprehensive update. *Orphanet Journal of Rare Disease.* Retrieved from https://ojrd.biomedcentral.com/articles/10.1186/s13023-020-01491-9

Hiort, O., Schütt, S., Bals-Pratsch, M., Holterhus, P., Marschke, C., & Struve, D. (2002, February 25). A novel homozygous disruptive mutation in the SRD5A2-gene in a partially virilized patient with 5alpha-reductase deficiency. *International Journal of Andrology.* Retrieved from https://pubmed.ncbi.nlm.nih.gov/11869378/

Ho, C. & Tan, H. (2013). Treatment of the hypogonadal infertile male-A review, Sexual Medicine Reviews. *International Society of Sexual Medicine.* 1(1), 42–49. Retrieved from: https://doi.org/10.1002/smrj.4

Hong, D. & Reiss, A. (2012). Cognition and behavior in Turner syndrome: A brief review. *Pediatric Endocrinology Reviews.* May 9, Suppl 2(02): 710–712.

Johnson, R.E. & Murad, M. (2009). Gynecomastia: Pathophysiology, evaluation, and management. *Mayo Clinic Proceedings.* 84(11), 1010–1015. doi: 10.1016/S0025-6196(11)60671-X

Jones, B.P., Williams, N., Saso, S., Thum, M-Y., Quiroga, I., Yazbek, J., Wilkinson, S., Ghaem-Maghami, S., Thomas, P., & Smith, J.R. (2018). Uterine transplantation in transgender women. *British Journal of Gynocology.* doi: 10.1111/1471-0528. Retrieved from: https://obgyn.

onlinelibrary.wiley.com/doi/pdf/10.1111/1471-0528.15438

Kruijver, P., Zhou, J., Pool, C., Hofman, M., Gooren, L., & Swaab, D. (2000). Male-to-female transsexuals have female neuron numbers in a limbic nucleus. *Journal of Clinical Endocrinology & Metabolism.* Retrieved from https://doi.org/10.1210/jcem.85.5.6564

Lanciotti, L., Cofini, M., Leonadri, A., Bertozzi, M., Penta, L., & Esposito, S. (2019). Different clinical presentations and management in Complete Androgen Insensitivity Syndrome (CAIS). *International Journal of Environmental Research and Public Health.* 16(7), 1268. doi: 10.3390/ijerph16071268

Lenders, N., McCormack, A., & Ho, K. (2020). Management of endocrine disease: Does gender matter in the management of acromegaly? *European Journal of Endocrinology.* Retrieved from https://eje.bioscientifica.com/view/journals/eje/182/5/EJE-19-1023.xml

Lipshultz, L., Ramasamy, R., & Armstrong, J. (2015). Preserving fertility in the hypogonadal patient: an update. *Asian Journal of Andrology.* 17(2), 197–200. doi: 10.4103/1008-682X.142772

Lucas-Herald, A., Bertelloni, S., Juul, A., Bryce, J., Jiang, J., Rodie, M., Sinnott, R., Boroujerdi, M., Lindhardt Johansen, M., Hiort, O., Holterhus, P.M., Cools, M., Guaragna-Filho, G., Guerra-Junior, G., Weintrob, N., Hannema, S., Drop, S., Guran, T., Darendeliler, F., ... Ahmed, S.F. (2016). The long-term outcome of boys with partial androgen insensitivity syndrome and a mutation in the androgen receptor gene. *The Journal of Clinical Endocrinology & Metabolism.* 101(11), 3959–3967. doi: 10.1210/jc.2016-1372

Ma, H., Marti-Gutierrez, N., Park, S., Wu, J., Lee, Y., Suzuki, K., Koski, A., Ji., D., Hayama, T., Ahmed, R., Darby, H., Van Dyken, C., Li, Y., Kang, E., Park, A., Kim, D., Kim, S., Gong, J., Gu, Y. ... Mitalipov, S. (2017). Correction of a pathogenic gene mutation in human embryos. *Nature*.

Melo, A., Ferriani, R., & Navarro, P. (2015). Treatment of infertility in women with polycystic ovary syndrome: approach to clinical practice. *Clinics (Sao Paulo)*. 70(11), 765–769. doi: 10.6061/clinics/2015(11)09. Retrieved from: https://www.ncbi.nlm.nih.gov/pmc/articles/PMC4642490

Nascimento, R., de Andrade Mesquita, I., Gondim, R., dos Apostolos, R., Toralles, M., de Oliveira, L., Cangucu-Campinho, A., & Barroso, U. (2018). Gender identity in patients with 5-alpha reductase deficiency raised as females. *Journal of Pediatric Urology*. 14(5). doi: 10.1016/j.jpurol.2018.08.021

National Institute of Diabetes and Digestive Kidney Disease. (n.d.). Acromegaly, 2020. Retrieved from www.niddk.nih.gov/health-information/endocrine-diseases/acromegaly

Nieschlag, E., Ferlin, A., Gravholt, C.H., Gromoll, J., Kohler, B., Lejeune, H., Rogol, A.D., & Wistuba, J. (2016). The Klinefelter syndrome: current management and research challenges. *Andrology*. Retrieved from https://doi.org/10.1111/andr.12208

O'Keefe, T. (1999). *Sex, gender & sexuality: 21ˢᵗ century transformations*. Extraordinary People Press.

Raziel, A., Friedler, S., Gidoni, Y., Ben Ami, I., Strassburger, D. & Ron-El, R. (2012). Surrogate in vitro fertilization outcome in typical and atypical forms of Mayer-Rokitansky-Kuster-Hauser syndrome. *Human Reproduction*.

27(1), 126–130. doi: 10.1093/humrep/der356

Regalado, A. (2018, April 20). Is it time to worry about human cloning again? *The Guardian.* Retrieved from: https://www.theguardian.com/lifeandstyle/2018/apr/20/pet-cloning-is-already-here-is-human-cloning-next

Reiner, W., & Gearhart, J. (2002, February 25). Discordant sexual identity in some genetic males with cloacal exstrophy assigned to female sex at birth. *The New England Journal of Medicine.* Retrieved from https://www.nejm.org/doi/full/10.1056/nejmoa022236

Richard-Eaglin, A. (2018). Male and female hypogonadism. *Nursing Clinics of North America.* 53(3), 395–405. doi: 10.1016/j.cnur.2018.04.006.

Stefanidis, K., Belitsos, P., Fotinos, A., Makris, N., Loutradis, D. & Antsaklis, A. (2011). Causes of infertility in men with Down syndrome. *Andrologia.* 43(5):353–357. doi: 10.1111/j.1439-0272.2010.01043.

Taneja, J., Ogutu, D., & Ah-Moye, M. (2016). Rare successful pregnancy in a patient with Swyer Syndrome. *Case Reports in Women's Health.* 121–2. doi: 10.1016/j.crwh.2016.10.001

Tartaglia, N., Davis, S., Hench, S., Nimishakavi, A., Beauregard, R., Reynorlds, A., Fenton, L., Albrecht, L., Ross, J., Visootsak, J., Hansen, R., & Hagerman, R. (2011). A new look at XXYY syndrome: Medical and psychological features. *American Journal of Medical Genetics Part A.* 146A(12), 1509–1522. Retrieved from https://www.ncbi.nlm.nih.gov/pmc/articles/PMC3056496/

Tartaglia, N., Howell, S., Sutherland, A., Wilson, R., & Wilson, L. (2010). A review of trisomy X (47,XXX). *Orphanet Journal of Rare Diseases.* doi: 10.1186/1750-1172-5-8

Thirumalai, A., Berkseth, K.E., & Amory, J.K. (2017). Treatment of hypogonadism: Current and future therapies. [version 1; peer review: 2 approved]. F1000Research 2017, 6(F1000 Faculty Rev):68 (https://doi.org/10.12688/f1000research.10102.1)

Uhlenhaut, N., Jakob, S., Anlag, K., Eisenberger, T., Sekido, R., Kress, J., Treier, A., Klugmann, C., Klasen, C., Holter, N., Riethmacher, D, Schutz, G., Cooney, A., Lovell-Badge, R. & Treier, M. (2009). Somatic sex reprogramming of adult ovaries to testes. *FOXL2 Ablation.* 139(6), 1130-1142. Retrieved from https://doi.org/10.1016/j.cell.2009.11.021

van der Horst, H., & de Wall, L. (2017). Hypospadias, all there is to know. *European Journal of Pediatrics.* Retrieved from https://pubmed.ncbi.nlm.nih.gov/28190103/

Varela-Cives, R., Méndez-Gallart, R., Estevez-Martínez, E., Rodríguez-Barca, P., Bautista-Casasnovas, A., Pombo-Arias, M., & Tojo-Sierra, R. (2015). A cross-sectional study of cryptorchidism in children: testicular volume and hormonal function at 18 years of age. *International Brazilian Journal of Urology.* 41(1): 57–66. Retrieved from https://www.ncbi.nlm.nih.gov/pmc/articles/PMC4752057/

Weidemann, W., Peters, B., Romalo, G., Spindler, K. D., & Schweikert, H. U. (1998). Response to androgen treatment in a patient with partial androgen insensitivity and a mutation in the deoxyribonucleic acid-binding domain of the androgen receptor. *The Journal of Clinical Endocrinology & Metabolism.* 83(4), 1173-1176. Retrieved from https://doi.org/10.1210/jcem.83.4.4704

Witchel, S. & Azziz, R. (2010). Nonclassic congenital adrenal hyperplasia. *International Journal of Pediatric Endocrinology.* doi: 10.1155/2010/625105

Yang, M., & White, P. (2017, February 13). Risk factors for hospitalization of children with congenital adrenal hyperplasia. *Clinical Endocrinology.* Retrieved from https://doi.org/10.1111/cen.13309

Yu, L., Wei, Y., Duan, J., Schmitz, D. A., Sakurai, M., Wang, L., Wang, K., Zhao, S., Hon, G. C., & Wu, J. (2021). Blastocyst-like structures generated from human pluripotent stem cells. *Nature.* Retrieved from https://doi.org/10.1038/s41586-021-03356-y

Zárate, S., Stevnsner, T., & Gredilla, R. (2017). Role of estrogen and other sex hormones in brain aging. Neuroprotection and DNA repair. *Frontiers in Aging Neuroscience.* doi: 10.3389/fnagi.2017.00430. Retrieved from https://www.ncbi.nlm.nih.gov/pmc/articles/PMC5743731/

Zhang, S., Zhu, D., Mei, X., Li, Z., Li, J., Xie, M., Xie, H., Wang, S. & Cheng, K. (2021). Advances in biomaterials and regenerative medicine for primary ovarian insufficiency therapy. *Bioactive Materials.* 6(7). 1957–1972. Retrieved from https://www.sciencedirect.com/science/article/pii/S2452199X20303339?via%3Dihub

Zhou, L., Gao, X., Wu, Y., & Zhang, Z. (2016). Analysis of pregnancy outcomes for survivors of the vanishing twin syndrome after in vitro fertilization and embryo transfer. *European Journal of Obstetrics & Gynecology and Reproductive Biology.* doi: 10.1016/j.ejogrb.2016.04.014

Chapter 3:
Gender Diversity and the Language Debate

Gender is seen as a social performance and construct, not a biological manifestation like sex. It is how you act out masculinity, femininity, both or neither. There is considerable importance in differentiating sex from gender for legal, social and relationships dynamics. Just as sex is physically variant and diverse, so is gender performance. When you move from space to space through time, your sex might not be changing but your gender performance can be interpreted differently according to varying social norms.

This is a concept you need to grasp when working with sex and/or gender diverse (SGD) groups in order to facilitate the individual's needs and not cause offence or harm. Do not expect other professionals to understand the difference nor indeed clients themselves at times, as unfortunately this concept is not generally included in educational curricula, even at medical schools and universities.

Gender diverse groups of people, other than stereotypically male or female roles, emerged in many cultures historically, dating back to Ancient Rome and Mesopotamian culture (Campanile et al., 2017; Ramet, 2002; Stryker, 2017; Roscoe, 1998). Native Hawaiians and Tahitians have had an intermediate gendered space called Māhū. There are other cultures that accept a broad spectrum of gendered spaces in their societies, like fa'afafine in Polynesia, four or five genders in Native American cultures, gender queer and non-binary in Western culture, drag queens, sworn virgins (women who live as men in Albania), Inuit third girl children who lived as men, Hijra in India, Aravani, Aruvani, Jagappa or Chhakka in Asia, kathoey or phuying prophet (a second kind of women) in Thailand and Mollies in historical England, who were effeminate gay men.

In fact, stereotypical exclusively masculine and feminine cultures only became prominent due to Judeo/Christian and Muslim fanaticism, colonisation and the eradication of diverse gender spaces due to religious and political puritanism. Indeed, the irony of Marxism is that in China, Russia and North Korea, gender became used to oppress people not to liberate them, particularly minorities. The same can be said for extremism in religions such as Christianity, Judaism and the Muslim faith where it overrode philosophical egalitarianism.

The confusion between sex and gender arises from the American political and legal evolution of the women's rights movement in the 1970s. Lawyers such as Ruth Bader-Ginsburg, in order to desensationalise the biased legal inequalities between the sexes, substituted the word "sex" with "gender" (Leder, 2018). This has led to cultural, legal, academic, medical and social confusion. Since English has been the major publishing scientific and research language in the West, the confusion further spreads to those who use English as a second language.

The confusion continues when we look at how English often does not translate well into other languages, cultural experiences or understandings around sex and gender. Since English was spread mainly as a Christian-based language, it carried with it the religious and social values of the countries of origin that were highly influenced by colonialism and conquered other cultures in an attempt to wipe out their social and linguistic experiences (Page & Sonnenburg, 2003). The problem is compounded further when a culture struggles to retain some of its values but has lost much of its linguistic independence, thereby losing its cultural understanding.

When one person is using the word "sex" when they are really referring to gender or vice versa, a healthcare professional may not understand what the client is trying to convey. Therefore, we as healthcare professionals must go to great lengths to unwind the client's true story.

We can see that many well-known females have lived as males including Saint Marinus who lived in a monastery as a Monk in the 6th century; James Gray, born in 1723 who joined the British Royal Navy fighting in battles; Peter Hagberg, born in Sweden in 1756, who also fought in battles; James Barry, born in the 1790s, a military surgeon in the British army who later became the Inspector General in charge of military hospitals; Albert Cashier, born in 1843, who fought in over 40 battles; Sammy Blalock, born in 1842, who fought as a soldier in the American Civil War; William Cathay born in 1844, who also fought in the American Civil War; Billy Tipton, born in 1914, an American saxophonist and jazz pianist who married and adopted children without his wife knowing his secret until he died (Setaysha, 2018); and Dante 'Tex' Gill, born in 1931 who was an American brothel and massage parlour owner who survived a bomb attack by the mafia in the 1970s (Revealed: The Incredible Life of Transgender Gangster, 2018).

Whether these people registered female at birth were cross-dressers, trans, transgender, transsexual or intersex is not for us to determine. What is clear is that, for at least part of their lives, they were male-identified personally, socially and could be professionally undetected as passing as men. They are part of gender diverse history, so much so that the actress Scarlett Johansson stepped down from playing Dante 'Tex' Gill in a proposed film in order to make room for a trans actor.

We also know that males passing as females has been common throughout human history: ancient Greek bronze statues from 700 BCE onwards depict male actors wearing women's clothes; Hippocrates, the ancient Greek physician, noted his observations of many eunuchs who preferred to speak, dress and act as women; in Elizabethan times in Shakespeare's plays, men dressed as females to play the female parts in theatrical productions; in China since the Yuan dynasty, men have dressed as women during the performance of Chinese opera; in Japan, men dressed as women in Kabuki theatre; Chevalier d'Éon, a French diplomat born 1728, dressed as female at court; and Stella and Fanny, born in 1847 and 1846, respectively, were a famous female impersonation double act in England who also dressed as women in the street (Garber, 1997; Bullough & Bullough, 1993). Registered males dressing as females were generally associated with entertainment, but females dressing as males were often associated with women liberating themselves beyond their social oppression (Devor, 1997).

Cultural experience of sex and gender diversity is important for us to understand when dealing with people from different cultures. Knowing those cultures helps us understand how we have constructed the limitations of our own understandings and how we might need to expand our knowledge.

The term **transgenderism** was originally used in the 1970s by Virginia Prince, an American male who lived as female but did not believe that sex realignment surgery was necessary (Prince, 2008). In fact, her views were so strong on the matter that they sometimes made her unpopular with people identifying as transsexual. In the 1990s, people started to come forward who felt the same about their experience, using the word 'transgender' to describe themselves. After around 2000, Americans began to use the word to mean all SGD groups who did not identify as intersex, which has caused enormous confusion in studying the different SGD groups due to linguistic conflation.

The confusion is compounded when people who are cross-sexed-identified differently from their natal registered birth undergo sex realignment and use the word 'transgender' to identify themselves; while other groups such as crossdressers also use the word to describe themselves. This throws up legal issues in sports classification and the rights to appropriate incarceration in the legal system. It has also caused problems within the women's rights movement where males who do not live as females want rights to female spaces, making many women feel unsafe. The confusion is further compounded when certain cultures and languages still use the word 'transsexual' to describing people who realign their sex.

Crossdressers/transvestites are people who adopt the dress of another sex part- or full-time but have no desire to be that sex. They are older descriptions but are often still used by some clients. Most crossdressers are part-time, and it may be a comfort reaction to stress or for sexual gratification (O'Keefe, 2007). Some may cross-dress full-time, living as a different gender but have no desire to be that sex. Many crossdressers are secretive about their dressing in private and a large proportion are heterosexual in heteronormative relationships.

Gender queer is very much a political term used in what is called the queer scene based around largely gay culture and what is often referred to as the LGBTIQ+ community. It can refer to non-normative gender presentation or even non-normative sexuality. The word "queer" used to be an insult meaning gay or lesbian but was reimagined by academia (queer theory) and street culture as a badge of honour for being a non-normative person (Johnston, 2015). It is hard to pin down what queer might mean because it is also used by heteronormative people who do not fit into society who consider themselves alternative (Lewis, 2015).

Gender non-binary is a phrase used by some people who try to pass through society as neither male nor female. They may not want to change their bodies from the original registered natal birth sex, but they wish to be considered socially neuter and may even seek to have documents that identify them as neuter (Rajunov & Duane, 2019).

Drag queens and kings are males who caricature dressing as females and vice versa, respectively, often for entertainment, as a political statement or because they like to dress that way. It is very much part of gay culture, particularly in older generations although television programmes like *RuPaul's Drag Race* have attained international fame (Dececco et al., 2014; Framke & Abad-Santos, 2018). While drag queens are associated with gay culture, there are heterosexual drag artists. It is also centred around defiance against oppression of these cultures and creating counter culture. Drag kings, however, have been almost exclusively associated with the lesbian culture (Halberstam & Volcano, 1999; Drysdale, 2019).

We can see in China today, as the gay culture pushes against the communist regime, the emergence of the drag scene and shows in gay clubs and bars. In Beijing, what started as a couple of charity events developed into drag shows that became a form of entertainment and tokenism against anti-gay oppression, as it has often done in the West (Ferrari, 2019).

Masculine females are women who are perceived and behave more masculine than commercialised images of how dainty and feminine women should be, according to societal norms. Those dainty perceptions are based on physiological, behavioural, social, work placement and political perspectives. From a feminist point of view, those stereotypical images of women are manipulations by patriarchy to control women and do not reflect the real experiences of being a woman, which are hugely varied according to need and circumstances

(Halberstam, 1998). Classifying women as masculine can also be seen as a misogynistic attempt to control women's sexuality. It would also be an incorrect assumption to presume that all masculine women are lesbians, intersex or trans.

Feminine males tend to come under more scrutiny in society than masculine females due to homophobia and male paranoia around a threat to men's masculinity. Males are generally more aggressive, driven by higher testosterone, show "rutting" behaviours and fraternity masculine peer evaluation of whether a male is "man enough" to be in their tribe. They are frequently comparing themselves to one another in judgment of how worthy they are to be considered male. Feminine males can be seen as weak and a threat to the pack.

This tends to put feminine males more at risk from violence and aggression in society than masculine females who are often referred to fondly as tomboys or an equivalent local colloquialism. Again, it is important not to read too much into social perceptions of feminine behaviour in males. If a male is atypically feminine, it does not mean they are gay, intersex or trans but rather they could simply be a variation of being male (Hill, 2007). They can be referred to as "sissy boys" and other derogatory labels but little research has been carried out into their life experiences, particularly heterosexual feminine males.

Native American cultures understand sex and gender differently according to their regions and tribes. These cultures had very fluid experiences of gender presentation and there was no absolute set of rules by which a person had to abide to be considered a gender, unlike invading European cultures. People who presented with cross-sex or gender male and female characteristics may be considered, even today, as two-spirit people, which was a blessing not a pathology. Tribes recognised up to five genders, with different terms in different languages; in Lakota, a feminine male is Winkté (male who behaves as a female); Niizh Manidoowag (two spirit) in Ojibwe; Hemaneh (half man, half woman) in Cheyenne; and many more names in other tribes. Since there are many different tribes, the meanings can change from tribe to tribe and there are some incorporated meanings of female-type male, male-type female, male and female, being gay, intersex or gender fluid (Williams, 2016).

Gender variance, need and tradition happens in some cultures and family situations when they are not able to economically or ecologically support too many people of one particular sex so changing a person's gender presentation was a form of survival adaption.

Third gender in Inuit culture saw that a girl child could be raised as a boy if there were too many girls in the family. If the family believed a child inherited the spirit of a dead relative of a different sex, the child could be raised as the opposite gender until puberty. Some may have become shamanic in adulthood and continued the third gender role (d'Anglure, 2005).

Fa'afafine (translation "in the manner of woman") in Samoa, American Samoa and the Samoan diaspora are males who identify themselves as having a third-gender/non-binary role. It is a uniquely traditional Samoan concept that is part of the culture, and they may appear as exaggeratedly feminine (Vanessa, 2007).

Fafatama is a further Samoan female-to-male description of third gender and again, it does not include the concept of being gay nor can it be translated into English. Like fa'afafine, fafatama are accepted and respected within the family as hard-working members of the community.

Albanian women who lived as men was a traditional cultural accommodation given when the males in a family all died then one of the women took on the role of the man, the head of the family, and dressed as a man and behaved as a man (Young & Eicher, 2001).

The Legal Re-Emergence of Gender Variance

Over the past 20 years, there has been a much greater legal recognition of gender variance, not specifically based on physiological sex, in different countries due to the efforts of civil rights campaigners. While more countries have been recognising the right of an individual who has undergone sex realignment from male to female and vice versa, so they change their documents, some countries are also recognising those outside of that category. This is not just the recognition of third gender but also of a wider gender spectrum that a person may experience and can include people who are inter-sex, trans or outside those categories who recognise their own social performance of a third or other gender.

In Germany (Oppenheim, 2019), people gained the right to be registered as a third sex, which allows people to be registered as "intersex" for those who do not fit the typical biological definition of male or female and have a doctor's certificate. The law change was heavily criticised by human rights campaigners for not going far enough to allow non-binary people to be registered as X or neuter. Since there is now evidence of possible genetic, hormonal, neurological and brain difference in non-official intersex people, that law may be challengeable for further extension under European human rights laws.

In Australia, it is also possible to have an elected X or other designations on a passport and some other documents. In 2014, Norrie May-Welby (SAGE co-founder) won the right in the High Court of Australia (HCA) to have "Sex Not Specified" on their documents after a failed sex alignment treatment that left them with a neuter identity (High Court of Australia, 2014). Some intersex individuals have also gained the right to have X on their documents. In Tasmania, a state of Australia, local politicians passed a law in 2019 (Humphries & Coulter, 2019) to allow sex or gender not to be put on birth certificates if the parents chose not to and also for all people over 16 to change their document status without parental permission.

Jamie Shupe achieved the right in Portland, USA to have their, at that time, non-gender status recognised (Dake, 2014). Later, they reoriented themselves back to living as male but the judgment remains the precedent for Americans achieving a non-gender status.

More countries have now recognised a sex and/or gender status that is other than male or female, but in many, it is a grey legal area or still a battle for recognition of the whole human sex and gender diverse spectrum. This constant battle and social denigration leads to greater minority stress, desperation, depression and elevated thoughts of suicide in these populations.

The Label Discourse

As healthcare professionals, we must learn to view the world through the clients' eyes. If you are not from a SGD group, this level of differentiation may make you dizzy at times, but its ethnographic comprehension will help you see your clients' unique world view. It is a basic principle of healthcare practice, called second position, where you try to see the world as the client sees it so you can understand how they need to negotiate their living terrain and journey, helping them avoid suicide.

If all you ever do as a clinician is see the world through your eyes, which is first position or a clinical objectivity (third position), you will never understand your client's world and will make endless mistakes in trying to help them. Objectivity only does not create empathy, but suffers from sympathy, which is what people on the verge of suicide do not need as it comes across as condescension and will destroy your rapport with your client.

We must still, however, as healthcare professionals, maintain the third position, seeing ourselves interacting with the client from a distance and from an objective perspective, while attempting to see the world through their eyes. Since these populations and sub-populations may be very foreign to you, you also need to keep an analytical perspective on the interactions between yourself and the client to be able to assess whether your interventions are working. Only viewing from your own perspective runs the risk of being misunderstood by the client, so change within the client's mental and emotional state might not take place.

For clinicians first coming into this field, negotiating the label wars is rather like trying to read a 1,000-digit binary code for the first time: It can be overwhelming. The complex profusion of labels, identities and medical and clinical classifications of different SGD groups and people is vast and neither is it static or black and white.

People become possessive of their self and group's descriptions. They invest their health, identities, emotions, politics, social beliefs, civil rights, connections to others and the world, and how they negotiate life, all via the way they describe themselves. When they perceive that other people do not respect or seem to understand those self-descriptions, clients can withdraw into the defensive fight or flight response, feeling threatened and breaking rapport.

Those from SGD groups have many different kinds of experiences. It is important to acknowledge those different experiences and the dynamics that affect a person's life. These different life dynamics lead to a variety of stressors and psychological drivers that can tip a client into the suicidal crisis. It is important for you as a healthcare professional dealing with these populations to familiarise yourself with the potential stressors for each group and individual, which may be leading the client to suicidal ideation.

Some people from intersex groups may have many short- or long-term medical problems that may require a range of surgeries and sometimes life-long medications, simply to sustain life. Other intersex people may have sex characteristics that are other than the average person, but they suffer from no medical side-effects so require no medical intervention. Having an identity or classification as intersex gives rights to medical care and misclassification as trans can, in some countries, threaten that right so those individuals can become very upset when described as trans.

Many intersex people may have had surgeries as a child without their permission to try and define them cosmetically as stereotypically male or female. Medical records and information of their biological history can also often be withheld from that individual unjustly. There are people who identify as strictly male or female even though they have intersex physical characteristics while other people with the same kinds of characteristics may identify as an intersex identity. There are people who even debate about whether the word "intersex" should be used at all. The fear around the word "sex" being conflated with gender for intersex people is about the erasure of intersex as a reality. The thrust of the intersexed movement is about empowering intersex people to make their own decisions about their own bodies and lives.

Many intersex campaigners take the position that people are born intersex. This is not the whole case as some people also become intersex during their life. Sex development is not purely intrauterine, genetic, embryotic or a foetal aberration. Sex development is lifelong and after birth people can masculinise or feminise through adrenal, pituitary and gonadal dysfunction, genetic variance or epigenetics, physical trauma, radiation, medication side effects, environmental toxicity and cancer.

It is noteworthy that many intersex people also deal with gender issues. If you were raised as one sex then transitioned, you also have to deal with gender reorientation. When claiming an identity as intersex, a person also has to negotiate the gender ramifications of how they are seen by others.

People who identify as transexed often consider themselves on the intersex spectrum but have also transitioned from their originally registered sex at birth. Again, some may have physical intersex characteristics but this is not necessarily the case. They also may undergo medical alteration of the body to become a sex that is other than the one they were registered at birth.

The word "transsexual" as a much older description was coined in the 1940s to describe people who transitioned from male to female or female to male via hormones and surgery. Older people still tend to use this word to describe themselves and in some cultures around the world, the term is still commonly used. The problem with this term is that it became used by psychiatry as a diagnosis of pathology to control patients and their life journeys, denying or granting them treatments they sought according to the clinician's whims, fancies and sometimes bizarre psychological theories. It also became used as a legal weapon to deny or grant people their civil rights. For this reason, it is less frequently used today.

Again, transitioning people may have difficulty reorienting their gender presentation in society. If you identify as one sex but are socially read as a non-coordinating gender, that can cause great emotional disturbance, depression and an increase in suicidal thoughts in some clients.

As mentioned earlier, the word "transgender" started life as a descriptive used by the American chemist Virginia Prince who used it to describe herself as someone who was registered male at birth but took hormones and lived as female. For many people who have transitioned from male to female or female to male, it is an unacceptable phrase and does not describe their experience. Indeed, to address them as such may be offensive.

Since that time, the word "transgender" has been adopted by many groups as a descriptive to identify themselves as other than strictly male or female or as a replacement for the old word "transsexual". The problem from a linguist perspective is that the term no longer describes a particular group of people who identify as cross-sexed or cross-gendered and disregards each group's individual dynamics, conflating one group's issues with another. We at Sex and Gender Education (SAGE) in Australia do not use "transgender" as an overarching descriptive as it becomes confusing when we campaign for a particular group's civil rights.

At SAGE we have one simple guideline that can help you stay up to date and allow you to have empathy with the client:

"How would you like me to address you?"

This may seem very simple, but it is highly effective because it immediately initiates respect for the client's experience. It dispenses with the opening question of, "What pronouns would you like me to use?". The client may ask you to use pronouns you have never heard of before like "Ze" or "Zi" or "Hir". To begin with, some pronouns may seem odd or cumbersome, but remember: a personal address is a form of respect for the other person's experience.

The use of the wrong pronoun or name can cause extreme offence and push the client into a defensive reaction when empathy is broken or damaged. We all accidently at times mislabel or misaddress people. In those instances, the best thing to do is to apologise immediately for your mistake, ask forgiveness and say you will do your utmost to get it right in future.

It is important to distinguish yourself from people who

purposefully use the wrong pronouns, address and descriptions of people from SGD groups. The client may have frequently suffered attacks from people who question their right to exist and dismiss the importance of addressing them correctly.

TERFs and SWERFs

It is wise to remember that many people from SGD groups are not privileged or middle-class. They may not have money, education, a career, work, housing and may be highly underprivileged, often living in a prejudicial society that does not support their existence and is even hostile towards them. On top of that, they constantly face attacks of all kinds.

Trans Exclusionary Radical Feminists (TERF) are members of an extreme branch of the women's movement that rejects and denies trans and other SGD groups' right to exist, particularly trans women (Serano, 2016). TERFs may be journalists, academics or extreme campaigners who seek to ban trans women and other SGD female-identified people from women's spaces.

TERFs constantly fail to understand the difference between intersex and trans and confuse the two. The tenet of their argument is that such people pose a threat to the sanctity of women's spaces, particularly lesbian spaces, though not exclusively, as some are heterosexual. They foster the illusion of a threat of violence, rape and the invasion of patriarchy, without being able to produce any real evidence of that happening en masse.

They can be aggressive, harassing, make diminutive comments, turn up at people's workplaces and march against trans people at pride parades to the extent that intersex and trans people are too afraid to attend again (Gabbatiss, 2018). Some write in newspapers and lecture at universities, hold conferences, all with the aim of turning women's society into unsafe spaces for female-identified people from SGD groups (Kaveney, 2012). They also have issues with people who began life as registered natal females who do not identify as female. However,

74

they can find little intellectual logic around their opposition to the person's choices. TERFism is akin to discrimination on grounds of religion and is an emotively-driven pathological obsession.

Many people from SGD groups, marginalised by society, turn to sex work in order to survive and pay for medical treatment (Nuttbrock, 2018); not thousands, but hundreds of thousands every year. This is often not even acknowledged by SGD campaigners who tend to lilac-wash our history into a middle-class struggle and omit those sex workers' history from academic studies.

Sex Workers Exclusionary Radical Feminists (SWERFs) espouse a branch of feminism that sees sex work for women as oppression and campaigns against its existence. It seems unable to address sex work for males, which includes millions of men. While it is true that the history of women has been and still is one of constant oppression, SWERFs fail to recognise that some women choose sex work, which is their right as free human beings. Eliminating sex work will not produce female emancipation, just another kind of oppression of women's choices.

SWERFs who demean women working in the sex industry are usually the same so-called feminists who are also TERFs. When you are a female-identified person working in the sex industry, the kind of attacks you receive from TERFs and SWERFs are constant, harassing and promote the social idea that you are a threat to society. This harassment and exclusion adds to the minority stress for people from SGD groups, pushing them further towards depression, substance abuse and living on society's margins, increasing suicidal thoughts.

The Public Abusers
Those who increase minority stress for SGD groups are not always those who harass, threaten, mislabel or attack them directly. They can be the lawmakers, politicians, religious

leaders, healthcare workers and academics who, without empathy, argue against the equal, full legal anti-discrimination protection for SGD groups that is automatically given to the rest of society. The harm they do in policy-making and public opinion can last for decades.

They use rhetoric like "a danger to society", "the possible collapse of the family unit", "end of moral guidance to our children" and a whole collective of doom-laden soundbites, none of which are supported by science or research. They are the purveyors of conservative puritanism, solely invested in the strictly male and female, Adam and Eve model of humanity.

They are obsessively and compulsively paranoid that the SGD groups are going to contaminate their gene pool; and frequently manoeuvre themselves into positions of great power and influence from which they seek to do as much damage as possible to the rights of SGD groups. They are as much a danger to the sanity of the suicidal SGD client as news of the end of the world.

The Prime Minister of Australia (at the time of writing), Scott Morrison publicly stated that he sent his daughters to a Baptist private school so they would not be exposed to information around sex that may be connected with SGD people (McGowan, 2018). Despite Australia having a Sex Discrimination Act that protects gay, intersex and gender diverse people against discrimination, Morrison voted against marriage equality for these groups of people.

In 2019, the Sultan of Brunei brought in an interpretation of Islamic laws or sharia that would see the death penalty for gay sex, which could have been used to murder SGD groups of people (Sultan of Brunei Drops Death Penalty for Gay Sex, 2019). After considerable public outcry, and boycotting of Brunei businesses led by Sir Elton John and the multi-million-dollar film star and businessman George Clooney, the Sultan eventually made a statement saying the law would not be enacted.

The Pope, during Pride month in 2019, made a declaration that being trans was wrong and that children who were somewhere between male and female should be, in the Vatican's opinion, normalised. A Vatican document stated that discussion in education about gender "destabilised the family unit" (Anonymous, 2019). This, of course, is from a misogynist institution that bans women from being priests. The article deeply upset many in the intersex and trans communities, some of whom were Catholics who felt betrayed and unsafe in the church. Hundreds of organisations publicly gathered together to urge the Vatican to reconsider.

In the USA, former President Trump incrementally revoked the rights of SGD groups of people in an effort to align himself with his largely Caucasian evangelical voters who are particularly anti-trans (Jones, 2018). The repeal of those rights included access to healthcare, access to public spaces, protection in prisons, and access to military service, many of which are covered in this text. The increase of minority stress in and sense of public hostility towards SGD groups clearly resembled the kind of public hysteria fostered in pre-Second World War Germany that led to so many deaths. Focusing on public hate and discontent toward SGD groups distracts the masses from the rich getting richer and the poor, in real terms, poorer.

The increase of attacks and murder of trans people in America since 2014, particularly trans women of colour, escalated to such an extent that the American Medical Association (AMA) was prompted to make a statement in 2019 to stem "the epidemic of violence against the transgender community, especially the amplified physical dangers faced by transgender people of color" (Ennis, 2019). The AMA voted to adopt a plan to bring attention to the issue. Board member Dr S. Bobby Mukkamala is quoted as saying: "Better data collection by law enforcement is needed to create strategies that will prevent anti-transgender violence."

In England and Wales, transphobic attacks have increased dramatically in recent years, trebling from 550 reports to 1,650 over the period examined from 2014 onwards. Almost half (46%) of these crimes in 2017–2018 were violent offences, ranging from common assault to grievous bodily harm (Marsh et al. 2019) While there are suggestions that better reporting may be partly responsible, monitoring organisations do suggest it is largely due to the rise of the new right-wing front on the streets.

It is important to be aware of the public gestalt in which the suicidal clients from an SGD group may be living and encounter on a day-to-day basis that increases and maintains their sense of minority stress.

Navigating that world as part of an extreme minority group can seem daunting as you have to continually explain yourself. When you add to that a sense of being unsafe in a frequently hostile world, for some, it becomes all too much to bear. We can support the client with our careful, articulate language or carelessly help push them over the edge to suicide with misdescriptions and the wrong addresses.

References

Anonymous. (2019, June 13). My Catholic, trans child is living proof of how wrong the Vatican is on gender. *The Guardian*. Retrieved from https://www.theguardian.com/commentisfree/2019/jun/13/catholic-trans-child-vatican-gender-transition-family

Bullough, V., & Bullough, B. (1993). Cross dressing then and now. *The Journal of Sex Research*. 30 (3): 289–291. doi:10.1080/00224499309551712

Campanile, D., Carlà-Uhink, F., & Facella, M. (2017). *Trans Antiquity: Cross-dressing and transgender dynamics in the ancient world* (1st ed). Routledge.

d'Anglure, B.S., (2005, November 1). The 'Third Gender' of the Inuit. *Sage Journals*. Retrieved from https://doi.org/10.1177/0392192105059478

Dake, L. (2016, June). Jamie Shupe becomes first legally non-binary person in the US. *The Guardian*. Retrieved from https://web.archive.org/web/20160616175106/ https://www.theguardian.com/world/2016/jun/16/ jamie-shupe-first-non-binary-person-oregon

Dececco, J., Sarria, J., & Gorman, M. (2014, January 2). *The empress is a man: Stories from the life of José Sarria.* (1st ed). United Kingdom: Routledge.

Devor, H. (1997). *FTM: Female-to-male transsexuals in society.* India University Press.

Drysdale, K. (2019, July 15). *Intimate investments in drag king cultures: The rise and fall of a lesbian social scene.* Palgrave Macmillan.

Ennis, D. (2019). American Medical Association responds to 'epidemic' of violence against transgender community. *Forbes*. Retrieved from https://www.forbes.com/ sites/dawnstaceyennis/2019/06/15/american-medical-association-responds-to-epidemic-of-violence-against-transgender-community/#247f7d34510b

Ferrari, C. (2019, April 16). Disco extravaganza: The drag scene in Beijing. *Culture Trip.* Retrieved from https://theculturetrip.com/asia/china/articles/ disco-extravaganza-the-drag-scene-in-beijing/

Framke, C., & Abad-Santos, A. (2018, March, 22). 11 moments that took RuPaul's drag race from scrappy underdog to pop culture behemoth. *Vox*. Retrieved from https://www.vox.com/culture/2018/3/22/17144202/ rupauls-drag-race-history-season-10

Gabbatiss, J. (2018). London Pride: Anti-trans activists disrupt parade by lying down in the street to protest 'lesbian erasure'. *Independent*. Retrieved from https://www.independent.co.uk/news/uk/home-news/anti-trans-protest-london-pride-parade-lgbt-gay-2018-march-lesbian-gay-rights-a8436506.html

Garber, M. (1997). *Vested interests: Cross-dressing and cultural anxiety*. Psychology Press.

Halberstam, J.. (1998). *Female masculinity* (1st ed). Press Books.

Halberstam, J., & Volcano, D.L. (1999). *The drag king book*. Serpent's Tail.

High Court of Australia. (2014). Registrar of Births, Deaths and Marriages v. Norrie, HCA 11.

Hill, D. (2007, March 1). "Feminine" heterosexual men: Subverting heteropatriarchal sexual scripts? *The Journal of Men's Studies*. Retrieved from https://doi.org/10.3149/jms.1402.145

Humphries, A, & Coulter, E. (2019, April 10). Tasmania makes gender optional on birth certificates after Liberal crosses floor. *ABC News*. Retrieved from https://www.abc.net.au/news/2019-04-10/birth-certificate-gender-laws-pass-in-tasmania/10989170

Johnston, L. (2015). Gender and sexuality I: Genderqueer geographies? *Sage Journals*. Retrieved from https://journals.sagepub.com/doi/10.1177/0309132515592109

Jones, S. (2018, October 28). Trump's alliance with evangelicals is at the heart of the White House's anti-transgender push. *Intelligencer*. Retrieved from http://nymag.com/intelligencer/2018/10/trump-evangelical-transgender.html

Kaveney, R. (2012, May 25). Radical feminists are acting like a cult. *The Guardian*. Retrieved from https://www.theguardian.com/commentisfree/2012/may/25/radical-feminism-trans-radfem2012

Leder, M. (2018). *On the basis of sex* [Motion picture]. Focus Features.

Lewis, H. (2016). *The politics of everybody: Feminism, queer theory, and Marxism at the intersection.* Zed Books.

Marsh, S., Mohdin, A., & McIntyre, N. (2019, June 15). Homophobic and transphobic hate crimes surge in England and Wales. *The Guardian*. Retrieved from https://www.theguardian.com/world/2019/jun/14/homophobic-and-transphobic-hate-crimes-surge-in-england-and-wales

McGowan, M. (2018, September 3). Scott Morrison sends his children to private school to avoid 'skin curling' sexuality discussions. *The Guardian*. Retrieved from https://www.theguardian.com/australia-news/2018/sep/03/scott-morrison-sends-his-children-to-private-school-to-avoid-skin-curling-sexuality-discussions

Nuttbrock, L. (2018). *Transgender sex work and society.* Harrington Park Press.

O'Keefe, T. (2007). *Autogynephilia and autoandrophilia in non-sex and gender dysphoric persons.* Paper presented at the World Association for Sexual Health conference, Sydney, Australia. Retrieved from https://tracieokeefe.com/autogynephilia-and-autoandrophilia-in-non-sex-and-gender-dysphoric-persons/

Oppenheim, M. (2019, January 1). Germany introduces third gender for people who identify as intersex. People who do not fit biological definition of male or female can now choose category 'diverse' on official documents.

The Independent. Retrieved from www.independent. co.uk/news/world/europe/germany-intersex-third-gender-identity-passport-lgbt-rights-a8706696.html

Page, M.E., & Sonnenburg P.M. (2003). *Colonialism: An international, social, cultural, and political encyclopedia* (Vol. 2). Santa Barbara, CA: ABC-CLIO.

Prince, V. (2008). Sex vs. gender. *International Journal of Transgenderism.* Retrieved from https://doi.org/10.1300/J485v08n04_05

Rajunov, M., & Duane, S. A. (2019). *Nonbinary: Memoirs of gender and identity* (1st ed). Columbia University Press.

Ramet, S.P. (2002). *Gender reversals and gender cultures: Anthropological and historical perspectives* (1st ed). Routledge.

Revealed: The incredible life of transgender gangster Mr Gill who controlled a criminal empire of brothels in 1970s Pittsburgh and will controversially be portrayed by Scarlett Johansson in her latest movie. (2018). *Daily Mail.* Retrieved from https://www.dailymail.co.uk/news/article-5924185/The-incredible-life-transgender-gangster-Mr-Gill.html

Roscoe, W. (2000). *Changing ones: Third and fourth genders in native North America.* Palgrave Macmillan.

Serano (2016). *Whipping Girl: A transsexual woman on sexism and the scapegoating of femininity.* Basic Books.

Setaysha, O. (2018). 10 women who lived their lives as men. *Stay at home mum.* Retrieved from https://www.stayathomemum.com.au/history/10-women-lived-lives-men/

Stryker, S. (2017). *Transgender history: The roots of today's revolution.* (2nd ed). Seal Press.

Sultan of Brunei drops death penalty for gay sex after backlash led by George Clooney and Elton John. (2019, May 5). *The Telegraph*. Retrieved from https://www.telegraph.co.uk/news/2019/05/05/sultan-brunei-drops-death-penalty-gay-sex-backlash-led-george/

Vanessa. (2007, August 27). *Memoirs of a Samoan, Catholic, and Fa'afafine*. United States: PublishAmerica.

Williams, T. (2016, June 19). Before European Christians forced gender roles, Native Americans acknowledged 5 genders. *Bipartisan Report*. Retrieved from https://bipartisanreport.com/2016/06/19/before-european-christians-forced-gender-roles-native-americans-acknowledged-5-genders/

Young, A., & Eicher, J. (2001, August 1). *Women who become men: Albanian sworn virgins (dress, body, culture)* (1st ed). Berg Books.

Chapter 4:
Research on the Occurrence of Suicidality in Sex and/or Gender Diverse Populations

We began this book by looking at the social-environmental world in which sex and/or gender diverse (SGD) groups live to begin our exploration of what drives some of those people to suicide. I began this project by trying to find out what research Sex And Gender Education (SAGE) Australia could contribute to the literature and the conversation. In looking at past research, I found how difficult this field is to research because access to participant groups was very limited since they were hard to reach en masse, frequently publicly unrecorded, did not respond well to calls to be involved in research and many did not want to run the risk of being publicity identified in any way.

Let us also consider that research is simply a photograph in time, recording what is observed and not necessarily what is true or enduring. The outcomes are determined by many factors including methodology, execution, scholastic constraints, participant willingness, participants and researcher confabulation, social permissibility, economic and resource limitations, legal acceptability, political colouration and the limitations of knowledge. For all of us as researchers, the usefulness of the knowledge we garner today may change tomorrow due to organisational and social evolution.

We also face the politically built-in obsolescence of research, in that quantitatively in the real world, it is driven by the five-year rule. The academic and drug company-driven pressure to produce research is often heavily propelled by the need to feed those industries over the reliability and validity of the research itself. If research is not seen as profitable, prestigious or favourable, or supports political policies in some way, it may not get funded or can be buried in the reference library. While we need research, we must also be its greatest critic, particularly when exploring marginal knowledge such as suicide in SGD groups and extend the five-year rule to take in older research.

The World Health Organization (WHO, 2019) reported that around a recorded 800,000 people carry out suicide every year, and it is the second-largest cause of deaths for people aged 15 to 29. Methods include imbibing poisons, inappropriate or large doses of medication, hanging, vein dissection, jumping off bridges and high structures, and placing oneself in situations of high risk and danger. One of the highest risks of successful suicide is a previous suicide attempt.

The Guardian (Australia's Rising Suicide Rate Sparks Calls, 2020) reported that government figures recorded 3,128 suicides in 2017 in Australia, an increase of 262 deaths from the previous year. Intentional self-harm moved from the 15th most common cause of death to the 11th in Australia, which was 12.6 deaths per 100,000. This crossed Australian cultures including Aboriginal and Torres Strait Islanders. The telephone mental health support service Lifeline received close to one million calls from callers experiencing mental health issues.

Many deaths due to suicide are not recorded as such, instead being listed as death by misadventure or accidental death. The evidence may be inconclusive or families may not want the suicide recorded on death certificates for religious or social reasons. The hidden figures for people who complete suicide from SGD groups are under-reported due to social stigma around SGD issues.

In this work, all sources considering suicide and suicidal thoughts in LGBTIQ+ communities were rejected and only papers on studies specifically studying suicidality in SGD groups of people were accepted. Papers and articles that studied suicide rates in gay, bisexual, lesbian, transgender, intersex and queer people as a collective population were considered an amalgamation of those groups, which does not give a true picture of suicide rates in SGD populations. Putting all of those groups together ignores that many of the samples would not be SGD but in fact heavily conflated with sexuality.

The current literature was also very unfocused in any particular direction. In taking early supervision on the research, I decided that the best way to add to the conversation was not to write another academic paper. Instead, this book aims to provide practical assistance for healthcare professionals helping people from SGD groups who have become suicidal; this was considered the better focus of our energies. Singular research would have strayed away from SAGE's remit, which is to promote the legal and human rights and dignity of people from SGD groups.

To give a clearer picture of the problem of suicide in SGD groups and what might be solutions to this, I sourced research and information from academic and clinical literature, grey literature, the media and the client group themselves individually to give a greater balance of knowledge. The sterility and doctoring of much academic research tends to give false impressions of people's actual existential experiences. It constantly misses the drivers of human behaviour and disregards the social circumstances in which those experiences occur.

We have to look at the occurrence and reasoning around suicide and suicidal ideation of people from SGD groups. There have been published studies in the past that have sought to collate information on the frequency of occurrence of suicidation in this population. However, these have often not attempted to profile deeper reasoning for the high levels of suicidal thoughts and successful suicides in SGD groups.

McNeil et al. (2012) published the *Trans Mental Health Study*, funded by the Scottish Government, which was coordinated

with public bodies, academics, community sector organisations and individuals to progress trans equality, human rights
and inclusion. It reported 48% of respondents to their self-
reporting survey had attempted suicide. Further, some 35%
had attempted suicide at least once, 25% more than once, 4%
thought about suicide every day and 3.2% were planning to take
their life. The researchers noted that before socially transitioning or changing their bodies, 63% of people did think about
suicide, though after transition that decreased dramatically to
3%. It was clear that the vast majority of those who experienced
suicidal thoughts believed it was connected with the difficulty
of being trans, from an SGD group and arising social issues.

An interesting point to highlight from this study encompassing the whole of the UK is the fact that many respondents
reported a reduction in suicidal thoughts after transition. This
study was also extremely thorough in giving respondents
choices on how to identify other than simply transgender.
However, it fell short in herding respondents to refer to their
experiences as gendered and not separating sex and gender
identification. In the UK, when someone transitions, it is sex
that is changed on birth certificates, not gender, even though
changing birth certificates for many SGD groups comes under
the *Gender Recognition Act.*

Haas et al. (2014) from the American Foundation for Suicide Prevention and the Williams Institute, UCLA School of
Law, USA, in the findings of the *National Transgender Discrimination Survey*, found 81.7% of respondents had seriously
thought about suicide during their lifetime and 40.4% had previously attempted suicide. The USA has one of the higher rates
of suicide in developed countries with an occurrence of 13.42
per 100,000 in 2016. People who detransitioned had higher
rates of suicide than those who did not detransition.

The researchers' analysis of the self-reporting survey (ages
19–89) stated that suicide attempts were further elevated

among multiracial (50.4%), Native American and Alaska Native (57.3%), lower educated (51.8%), lower socio-economic (56%) and 18–24 years old (45%) populations. Those that disclosed their sex and gender status to everyone were generally more susceptible to suicide because of more exposure to discrimination, causing a higher level of minority stress.

The suicide attempts in trans men was 46% and 42% trans women. Those who identified as crossdressers assigned male at birth but who intermittently dressed as female was the lowest group at 21%, probably due to enjoying male privilege in most of their daily lives. Other life circumstances measured included HIV status (51%), disabilities (55–65%), physical conditions (56%), mental health conditions (65%), harassed and bullied at elementary school (50%), experienced refusal by healthcare practitioners to treat them (60%), sexual assault at college (78%), sexual assault at school (69%), experienced discrimination by police personnel (61%) and sexual violence by police officers (60–70%).

While the study was quite comprehensive, it was called "Suicide Attempts among Transgender and Gender Non-Conforming Adults", and its sub-title was "National Transgender Discrimination Survey". Again, this poorly defines those populations and may not include many individuals who are intersex, when many intersex people have transitioning experiences, as do SGD groups who do not identify as transgender. Haas, Rodgers and Herman also found that:

"There was an observed strong differential on family dynamics and suicide attempts: a lower-than-average prevalence of lifetime suicide attempts (33%) was found among respondents who said their family relationships had remained strong after coming out. In contrast, the prevalence of suicide attempts was elevated among respondents who reported experiencing rejection, disruption, or abuse by family members or close friends because of anti-transgender bias."

Many of these observations could be paralleled across cultures and even sub-cultures, showing often-experienced commonalities, like rejection by families, educational exclusion, social ostracisation, economic disadvantage and harassment and violence from law enforcement. Such experiences for people from SGD groups are a frequent reality a great deal of the time in all countries.

Costa and Colizzi (2016) reviewed studies on the application of cross-sex hormones and better mental health outcomes. They found that:

"Inclusion criteria for studies were as follows:
1) studies in gender dysphoria,
2) studies investigating the mid/long-term effects of cross-sex hormonal treatment, and
3) studies measuring mental health-related parameters, including
    a) depression
    b) anxiety
    c) personality
    d) quality of life
    e) dissociative symptoms
    f) psychopathology
    g) psychosocial/emotional functioning
    h) distress, and
    i) self-esteem

Exclusion criteria were as follows:
1) studies in which cross-sex hormonal treatment was not the intervention of interest (i.e., studies including cross-sex hormonal treatment only as a confounder/covariate of no interest) and
2) studies in which the mental health-related outcomes were not directly reported upon."

Their findings suggest that in most studies, although not all, gender dysphoria-related distress (and presumably sex dysphoria) may be relieved by the administration of voluntary cross-sex hormones. In some studies, there was a different balance between the benefits for male-to-female and female-to-male transitioning patients, with male-to-female patients experiencing a greater reduction in anxiety.

This partly supports what has long been reported by many people experiencing sex and/or gender dysphoria. Less distress does equal less risk of suicide, particularly when dealing with individuals who are pre-transition, do not have access to care or who feel life is too intolerable without transition.

Again, however, it is important to remember that each case is an individual who brings with them a set of their own psycho-dynamics, strengths and in some cases psychopathologies. In the case of undetected, unexplored or unmanaged psychopathologies like schizophrenia, borderline personality disorder, bipolar or dissociative disorders, prior to administration of hormones, outcomes may be less favourable.

Virupaksha et al. (2016) found that elevated suicide rates and attempts in India were higher than the general populations in a group that they labelled as transgendered people. They did not, however, clearly define transgender people. Their literature searches included five behavioural databases and grey literature that suggested incidence rates of 32% to 50% across a number of countries. In India, 50% attempt suicide before their 20th birthday, but we need to note that it is impossible to estimate the true rate of completed suicide due to India's poor data collection figures. Virupaksha et al. contended that:

"Gender-based victimization, discrimination, bullying, violence, being rejected by the family, friends, and community; harassment by intimate partner, family members, police and public; discrimination and ill treatment at healthcare

systems are the major risk factors that influence the suicidal behavior among transgender persons."

While this meta-analysis looks at deeper reasoning from the literature about why transgender people became suicidal, it failed to precisely quantify the parameters of the source groups. The term "Hijra" cannot be translated into the Western term 'transgender' as both are exclusive experiences. Many Hijra do not identify as transgender in India and vice versa. It also refers to the transgender community, but there are people who identify as transsexual in India who are not part of any of those communities. Such communities are not transgender communities within the Western sense but rather Hijra families by choice. Their dynamics are considerably different from Western-sourced studies, therefore creating different psychodynamics individually and in intragroup relations.

Jones et al. (2016) published an independent, self-reporting study including stories and statistics of 272 self-identified intersex Australians. Of the respondents, 19% reported having attempted suicide, 26% had self-harmed, 42% had thoughts about self-harming and 60% had thoughts about suicide directly relating to their sex variances. The average Australian suicide rate was far lower at 3%.

Notably, this study indicates high rates of poverty reported by the majority of participants, with 63% earning an income under AU$41,000 per year and 41% earning less than AU$20,000 per year (the minimum wage during the survey period was AU$34,158. This shows a large percentage weighted towards national poverty levels. Heflin and Iceland (2009) clearly link the relationship to higher levels of depression, poverty and material hardship in lower socioeconomic groups, which will naturally lead to higher levels of suicide.

Intersex people may be born with obvious primary and secondary sex characteristics, clearly different from stereotypically male or female children, but others discover or develop their sex differences later in life. Stressors that affect this population may be enforced surgery or involuntary medical treatments, lack of appropriate medical help, poverty and the burden of continuing medical costs, physical difficulties engaging in sex, infertility, stigma, lack of social acceptance, lack of positive social reinforcement, bullying, subjection to violence, isolation, family rejection, difficulty with relationships, inability to work due to medical complications, mental health issues and discrimination.

Some problems with the study, however, are that many intersex people do not know they are intersex, on discovery become stealth (trying not to be seen), are not told the true extent of their intersex, do not identify as intersex or are intersex people who are happy with the treatment they received as children; therefore, they might not respond to such studies.

This small sample of Australian intersex people was 272 out of what must be at least 250,000-plus, which is the minimum of 1% of the population. This renders the study as only reporting on those intersex people who identify as intersex, not those who are intersex but identify as typical males or females, who may or may not be in the higher socio-economic groups, adjusting to an ordinary life.

During the debate of the California bill to ban medics from performing unnecessary surgeries and procedures on intersex children, the California Medical Association and Societies for Pediatric Urology both opposed the ban (Gutierrez, 2019). They reasoned that the law should not dictate medical decisions; however, they were compromised in their opposition because they had a financial self-interest. The bill was asking for unnecessary and non-life-threatening medical decisions and surgeries to be delayed until the child themselves could decide what they wanted for their bodies.

It is important to consider that medicine frequently hides

intersex conditions and realities from the public and patients themselves so those patients often do not show up in the statistics. Much of the medical establishment's obsession with normalising intersex people's bodies focuses on pathologically attempting to eliminate intersex from the human equation, characterising it as being shameful and improper, and shrouding it from view.

Adams et al. (2017) carried out a meta-analysis of a selection of US and Canadian grey literature from the WorldCat database, checked against Google Scholar, reporting transgender suicidality in papers and articles between 1997 and 2017. The 42 studies reviewed on average showed that 55% of respondents and participants reported suicidal ideation and 29% had attempted suicide in their lifetime. Suicide ideation was higher in those registered male at birth who transitioned to female, while suicide attempts occurred more frequently in those who were registered female at birth and transitioned to male.

While these figures appear alarming, it is important to consider that many of these studies will have used single-source reporting, such as self-reporting questionnaires, so their reliability must be viewed with caution. They are also subjected to linguistic and cultural distortion, altered and changed interpretations according to the social attitudes and laws of the places where the studies were carried out. What it means to be intersex, trans, neuter or bi-gendered in one culture is never the same in another culture. It is quantitively impossible to adjust for those variables en masse because too many constantly shifting variables are involved.

Strauss et al. (2017) conducted the *Trans Pathway Survey*, an online survey of Australian trans youth and their mental health, in 2016, with the 2017 publication funded by the Western Australian Government. The survey analysed the reported experiences of 14–25-years-olds in accessing mental health and medical services and drivers of poor mental health. It included a wide range of people who identified as intersex, people who were unsure if they were intersex or not, transgender-identified persons and people who were gender-questioning or fluid. It included 859 participants. Trans youth were from SGD groups of people and 194 were parents and guardians.

The study found 48.1% of SGD respondents had attempted suicide at least once. This was 14.6 times greater than the general Australian populous. At the time of the study, 70.04% reported having been diagnosed with depression; 72.2% had been diagnosed with anxiety: 25.1% with Post-Traumatic Stress Disorder; 61% were feeling isolated from mental health and medical services; 42.1% had reached out to service providers that they believed did not understand, respect or have previous experience with gender diverse people; 78.9% had issues with school, tertiary education and university; 68.9% suffered discrimination; 65.8% had a lack of family support; 22% faced accommodation issues or homelessness; 89% experienced peer rejection; and 74% experienced bullying. Notably, this study could probably be easily reproduced in many Western cultures.

While discrimination laws in Australia at the time of the study were quite comprehensive, the results indicate they failed to a large extent to protect people from SGD groups from discrimination that is fuelled by ignorance in medicine, education and public and religious extremism, where legal loopholes existed.

Zeluf et al. (2018) published a self-selecting, online survey of victimisation and suicidal thoughts of Swedish trans people. Of the 796 trans respondents, aged between 15–94, 37% reported serious thoughts of suicide during the 12 months prior to the survey and 32% had previously attempted suicide. Of the respondents, 19% reported having been exposed to trans-related violence; 52% exposed to trans-related offensive behaviour in the previous three months; and 64% reported living in fear of discrimination. Experiencing offensive behaviour during the previous three months and lifelong experiences of violence were significantly associated with suicidality. Reduced quality social interactions and lack of support were also associated with increased suicidal thoughts. Compared to other Swedish studies reporting on the general population, it is evident that the risk factors for trans people moving to suicidation were more than seven times the national average.

The authors reported that, in Sweden, successful suicides among SGD people post-transition gender-affirming surgery, who were registered a different sex at birth, was elevated compared to the general population. Also, Swedish studies on trans suicide tended to focus on individuals who identified as having experienced gender dysphoria and did not generally consider non-binary or gender-fluid individuals who may also experience victimisation and discrimination. While Sweden has anti-discrimination laws designed to protect SGD groups of people, discrimination still takes place and individuals report they can find it difficult at times to get the treatment they believe they need from nationally-financed sex and/or gender identity clinics.

Toomey et al. (2019) gathered data from Student Life: Attitudes and Behaviors survey, published in the *American Journal of Pediatrics*, of adolescents aged between 11–19 from 2012–2015. Nearly 14% of adolescents reported attempted suicides, although children transitioning from female to male suicided the highest rate (50.8%); those identifying as not strictly male or female came next (41.8%); followed by those transitioning from male to female (29.9%). This was comparative to heteronormative adolescent females (17.6%) and males (9.8%).

The problem with this self-reporting study is that it is not longitudinal. In adolescence, many people who are questioning their masculinity or femininity are also questioning their sex and gender self-image. For many, this questioning changes after adolescence as they move into the adult years, the breeding cycle of their lives, and are faced with the harsh reality of surviving in a stereotypical industrialised workplace and society. However, the study does contribute the conclusion that suicide prevention in such populations could be enhanced by paying attention to variability within those populations.

In considering the literature, and this is only a small sample, we have to consider more closely what it can and cannot tell us. Certainly, we need quantitative research, but what it can tell us about these populations is extremely limited and often unreliable with low validity.

Firstly, academia has generally divided the populations into two distinct groups: intersex and transgender. It is important to remember that intersex is a far bigger group than simply those who have been born with ambiguous genitalia or the strict parameters that many intersex campaigners wish to put around the label of intersex.

The confusion around the label "transgender" and who or what it includes has made it impossible to quantitatively study groups like those who identify as transexed, transsexual, gender-fluid or non-binary because people responding or being involved in research around being transgender takes in too many sub-groups.

Also, quantitative research works best when it studies very narrow concepts, constructs or phenomena, where variables are well defined. The wild variables in all studies around suicide in people from SGD groups are interpersonal relationships and social attitudes, both of which 99% of researchers ignore or are ignorant of. These highly influential wild variables render much of the research unreliable and invalid, even though it has passed academic rigour, as it fails to take account of the realities of the world in which SGD groups live.

Bonierbale et al. (2016) carried out a study of 108 French transsexuals, 18 years and older, using the Minnesota Multiphasic Personality Inventory 2 (MMPI-2). The study was carried out at a psychiatric unit of a major public hospital where the participants were part of a program for, what was described as, a standardised sex reassignment procedure, with a median age of 31, 50% applying for male to female transition and vice versa. The team were screening for the presence of psychopathology, which it was proposed may reveal the linked psychopathology of all individuals applying for such processes. The initial sample was larger but after testing, some were considered not suitable for sex reassignment surgery and classified as invalid tests. The screening was carried out by both a psychiatrist and psychologist, and patients had to agree to gain referrals for surgery.

Notably, this study takes place in complete social isolation. France has a deeply patriarchal medical system that has always acted as an overbearing gatekeeper to allowing people to transition through the public medical system. Traditionally, transsexuals in France have frequently lied in those programs about themselves and have passed on stories of how to tell clinicians what they want to hear to get referrals. In France, being transsexual still carries great stigma, blocking work and social opportunities.

We can see in Paris that several hundred trans women work in the Bois de Boulogne park area as sex workers, which is 80% of the sex workers there, because they have problems getting work (*France 24*, 2017). While it has become legal to sell sexual services in France, it is illegal to buy them. This has put considerable pressure on the sex worker population and made them subject to more frequent violent attacks, disappearances and murders. Some sex workers say they have stopped calling the police because they seem not interested. Even though they carry pepper spray and tasers, many will not work late into the night for the fear of danger, so they live with the constant fear of attack and are on high alert every time they are at work.

The MMPI 2 may have been adjusted for the French population but not for subgroups like transsexuals and not for smaller subgroups like those who use private, non-state medical and sometimes black-market help for fear of rejection and prejudice. In reality, such people should register high for paranoia and fear on an MMPI 2 and that would be normal for them because of social stigmatisation and oppression. Many of those sex workers working in the Bois de Boulogne and other areas, however, are illegal immigrants and would not qualify to access the public medical systems. Therefore, they are marginalised and live on the edge of society, encountering depression and minority stress.

We also have to ask ourselves the sociological questions of would women being screened for an abortion, tubal ligation, hysterectomy, mastectomy due to cancer risk and men having a vasectomy be screened with the MMPI 2? Screening SGD groups under the pretence that knowing about any psychopathologies would enable better treatment outcomes assumes psychopathology in the first place. So, not only does this enforced study not have reliability or validity, but the very process is an abuse of power and institutionalised transphobia that increases the risks of depression and suicide.

While the media constantly quotes research around suicide in SGD groups to support a storyline or fulfil a political agenda, it is unaware of or ignores its scientific failings. Scientists and policymakers also quoting the research are frequently citing poorly-sourced information.

There are few quantitative research-based pull quotes in the media to rely on when it comes to suicide rates in people in SGD groups because so much of the research is unreliable. The groups and sub-groups are at times quite different in their experiences, physically, mentally and socially, and to try and study them or help them as one homogenous population involves considerable structural problems.

For us as healthcare professionals seeking true sources of information around suicide in SGD populations, we need to garner qualitative information. This is because we must treat each case as an individual, considering the influence of the person's psychodynamics, familial and social circumstances. In this work, therefore, we will pay great attention to individual cases, which gives us far more information on the people from SGD groups experiencing suicide.

In our consideration of the research, we consider the ethics of working with and how we work with SGD groups who experience suicidal ideation. As healthcare professionals, we have to negotiate several ethical filters to arrive at decisions on treatment and help to create health plans with our clients. Those filters include the law, the codes of ethics in our own particular professional associations, specialist standards of care for particular groups and subgroups, and consideration of the human rights of the client in accordance with expected international standards. At times, some of the ethics will be conflicting and we will have to make educated and judgment calls based on the best interests of our clients.

Fisher et al. (2016) acknowledged that clinicians face major dilemmas when attempting to assign and reassign gender (and presumably sex) for children born with Disorders of Sex Development (DSD). However, their suggestion of an international registry of people with DSD is somewhat disturbing and intrusive on patients' privacy.

Research on guidelines for treating people with DSD, or being intersex, is currently a moving target and evolving field. The controversy is divided into the two distinct fields of functional and remedial cosmetic medicine. Functional approaches require medical intervention to support life. The cosmetic approach is to change the non-medical emergency—that is, the body of the child or person—to normalise them into male or female as much as possible. Most people accept that medical intervention when a child or adult experiences a physical life-threatening condition is acceptable.

The controversy that has arisen is that many people who underwent involuntary medical intervention as children, when their life was not in danger, are unhappy with the outcomes, which can lead to lack of sexual satisfaction, at times the wrong assignment of sex and gender, depression and even suicidal ideation. Such dissatisfied intersex people seek to prevent doctors in future from intervening on the child's behalf without the child's permission. Instead, doctors should only do so when the child is educated about what they would like to happen to their body.

Carpenter (2018) wrote in the *Journal of Reproductive Health Matters:* "Intersex people and bodies have been considered incapable of integration into society." This has been true within Western Medicine and some native cultures. Some cultures, however, had spaces and traditionally accepted intersex people, like Native American and Indonesian cultures before Westernised bioethics of religious extremism sought to eliminate traditional values. Ethically, we need to learn from those cultures and allow intersex children and people to be able to make sex and gender assignment decisions based on their own wishes. They may at times not see being intersex as a disorder of sex development and forcing that label on them can lead to lower levels of patient dissatisfaction, depression and suicide.

Bizic et al. (2018) reviewed the bioethics around the treatment of people who experienced what they called gender dysphoria (which would also include those who experience sex dysphoria in trans groups). Their review looked at gender reassignment (often commonly known as sex affirmation), the provision of hormones, surgery, social stigma, the need for legal recognition and the application of such treatment to youth groups. They quoted the *DSM 5* (American Psychiatric Association, 2013) occurrence figures of gender dysphoria for adult natal males (0.005–0.014%) and adult natal females (0.002–0.003%), which do not coordinate with some of the studies I have reviewed. Only 10–20% were children, some of whom did not cross-sex identify to their registered natal birth, in coming into adolescence.

Two distinct themes came out of Bizic et al.'s research. They recognised that even when employing a multi-disciplinary approach, and adhering to ethical treatment guidelines, not all treatments delivered satisfactory outcomes. A number of patients reviewed regretted transition and were attempting to revert to their original registered birth sex. Secondly, they identified poor outcomes with inadequate social adaptation, psychiatric comorbidity, poor psychological evaluation prior to transition and dissatisfaction with physical, aesthetic or functional outcomes. This suggests the need for higher levels of psychotherapeutic help for patients considering transition, both pre- and post-transition, to improve patient outcomes including a reduction in suicidation.

The field of working with people who do not fit the exclusive male or female paradigm is so far largely quantitatively and qualitatively under-researched. People in these groups may be intersex, transgender, queer, sex non-specific, gender non-specific, gender-fluid identified or a whole host of descriptions that may have traditional cultural interpretations that are other than male or female. What is important to remember when dealing with clients from these groups is that they are the margins of the margins of society. They are small subgroups of the SGD spectrum and attract little or no research funding, and so we rely on anecdotal, ethnographic and anthropological reporting of their experiences. This was the case with Ramet's (1996) examination of the eradication of gender-fluid social spaces through the invading colonisation of European cultures.

All SGD groups, and some in particular, experience minority stress at times, leading to depression and suicidal ideation. This is especially true for some sub-groups, as they will stand out more in society than other SGD groups who blend more into male and female social roles. This means that many from these groups are never stealth and can be highly visible and frequently targeted for social and violent attacks. Also, these groups often do not have the right to documents that reflect their identity or have legal protection against discrimination.

Working with children is the area raises the most controversy and criticism from extreme right-wing conservatives in medicine and politics who are invested in the solely male and female, heteronormative, polarised sex and gender perspectives of human existence. They are frequently driven by religious extremism that fails to accept the pluralism of humanity and nature. Groups like the American Academy of Pediatrics (2018) support children finding and living their own sex and gender identities. Opposing groups, however, like the American College of Pediatrics' President Dr Michelle Cretella (2017), are largely against children being allowed to live in roles other than natally registered male or female at birth and see carers that allow it as abusive, and clinicians' actions who sanction it as malpractice. Dr Cretella specifically sees sex and gender diversity as a mental illness.

Children who experience sex and/or gender dysphoria can become highly distressed and frustrated about their situation and do attempt suicide and at times succeed to suicide, particularly if they experience ostracisation and bullying.

Research on suicidality in children who are intersex is virtually non-existent and understudied, possibly largely because many intersex children do not know they are intersex and being intersex is shrouded in such secrecy. Adult qualitative reporting demonstrates that many intersex adults talk about how traumatising it was for them as children and how they did consider and even attempt suicide.

Suicide attempts in trans children is far more widely researched. Olson et al. (2018) reported low levels of psychopathology in young adults who socially transitioned as transgender children. What we see later in this volume, however, is that children from SGD groups who do not feel supported in their sex and gender affirmation or respected do attempt and succeed to suicide.

We must always keep in mind the safety and wellbeing of the individual patient/client. The research may give us some indications of suicide risk in SGD groups, but it may also mislead us. In aiding those children and people, we must always be mindful of the mental state of the individual client and factor in any minority stress they may be experiencing that could lead to suicide.

Australia allows people to choose male, female or X on their passports and documents. Birth certificates may state male, female or sex non-specific and moves are in place by campaigners to remove sex status from birth certificates altogether. So, legally, people could present as whatever sex or gender they wish and be protected by the *Sex Discrimination Act* against harassment.

The problem sociologically and historically is that many gender diverse people often do not have biological roots for their behaviour, although some may, so they end up in legal grey spaces. We also need to consider anthropologically that the semantics and pragmatics of language plus cultural perspectives often lead to the meaning of that human experience not being strictly translated into different languages or cultural interpretations.

Some people may not be happy with their social gender role performance and presentation and experience gender dysphoria. It may be uncomfortable for them, and they may not feel they can fulfil those gender expectations associated with their assigned biological sex. Other people are gender diverse and may not experience gender dysphoria but may simply wish to act out a different gender performance than their assigned biological sex.

Some people may experience sexuality dysphoria and not be happy with their sex act impulses and the people they are driven to have sex with (O'Keefe, 1999). They may wish to try and alter their sexual impulses through various kinds of physical or psychological therapies. Here we cross over into the area where a small group of people whose sex and gender identity may be driven by impulses connected to their sexuality, such as erotic crossdressing, autogynophilia and autoandrophilia (O'Keefe, 2010). This is not the case for most SGD diverse groups, but the assumption that it is creates chronic minority stress for many people from SGD groups.

References

Adams, N., Hitomi, M. & Moody, Cherie. (2017). Varied reports of adult transgender suicidality: Synthesizing and describing the peer-reviewed and Gray literature. *Transgender Health.* Retrieved from https://www.ncbi.nlm.nih.gov/pmc/articles/PMC5436370/

American Academy of Pediatrics. (2018). *AAP policy statement urges support and care of transgender and gender-diverse children and adolescents.* Retrieved from https://www.aap.org/en-us/about-the-aap/aap-press-room/Pages/AAP-Policy-Statement-Urges-Support-and-Care-of-Transgender-and-Gender-Diverse-Children-and-Adolescents.aspx

American Psychiatric Association. (2013). *Diagnostic and statistical manual of mental disorders.* (5th ed.). Washington, DC: Author.

Australia' s rising suicide rate sparks calls for national target to reduce deaths. (2020, September 26). *The Guardian.* Retrieved from https://www.theguardian.com/australia-news/2018/sep/26/australias-rising-suicide-rate-sparks-calls-for-national-target-to-reduce-deaths

Bizic, M. R., Jeftovic, M., Pusica, S., Stojanovic, B., Duisin, D., Vujovic, S., Rakic, V. & Diordievic, M. L. (2018). Gender dysphoria: Bioethical aspects of medical treatment. *Biomed Research International.* doi: 10.1155/2018/9652305

Bonierbale, M., Baumstarck, K., Maquigneau, A., Gorin-Lazard, A., Boyer, L., Loundou, A., Auquier, P. & Lançon, C. (2016). MMPI-2 profile of French transsexuals: The role of sociodemographic and clinical factors. A cross-sectional design. *Scientific Reports.* doi:10.1038/srep24281

Carpenter, M. (2016). The human rights of intersex people: addressing harmful practices and rhetoric of change. *Taylor & Francis Online.* Retrieved from https://doi.org/10.1016/j.rhm.2016.06.003

Costa, R. & Colizzi, M. (2016). The effect of cross-sex hormonal treatment on gender dysphoria individuals' mental health: a systematic review. *Neuropsychiatric Disease and Treatment.* doi: 10.2147/NDT.S95310

Cretella, M., (2017). *Transgenderism: A mental illness is not a civil right.* Retrieved from https://www.youtube.com/watch?v=s57T27M1ZXk [appears to have been removed]

Fisher, A.D., Ristori, J., Fanni, E., Castellini, G., Forti, G. & Maggi, M. (2016). Gender identity, gender assignment and reassignment in individuals with disorders of sex development: a major of dilemma. *Journal of Endocrinological Investigation, 39*(11), 1207–1224.

France 24 [English]. (2017, September 8). *Transsexual prostitutes in Paris face increasing violence.* Retrieved from https://www.youtube.com/watch?v=dj1cooYHkwU

Gutierrez, M. (2019, April 8). Bill to ban cosmetic genital surgeries on intersex infants delayed. Doctors opposed it.

The Los Angeles Times. Retrieved from https://www.latimes.com/politics/la-pol-ca-intersex-genital-surgery-20190408-story.html

Haas, A. P., Rodgers, P. L. & Herman, J. L. (2014). Suicide attempts among transgender and gender non-conforming adults. Findings of the National Transgender Discrimination survey. Retrieved from https://williamsinstitute.law.ucla.edu/wp-content/uploads/AFSP-Williams-Suicide-Report-Final.pdf

Heflin, C. M., & Iceland, J. (2009). Poverty, material hardship and depression. *Social Science Quarterly,* (90)5, 1051–1071. doi: 10.1111/j.1540-6237.2009.00645.x

Jones, T., Hart, B., Carpenter, M., Ansara, G. Leonard, W. & Lucke, J. (2016). Intersex: Stories and statistics from Australia. *Open Book Publisher.* Retrieved from https://interactadvocates.org/wp-content/uploads/2016/01/Intersex-Stories-Statistics-Australia.pdf

McNeil, J., Bailey, L, Ellis, S., Morton, J. & Regan, M. (2012, September). *Trans mental health study.* Scottish Transgender Alliance. Retrieved from https://www.scottishtrans.org/wp-content/uploads/2013/03/trans_mh_study.pdf

O'Keefe, T. (1999). *Sex, gender & sexuality: 21st century transformations.* Extraordinary People Press.

O'Keefe, T. (2007). *Autogynephilia and autoandrophilia in non-sex and gender dysphoric persons.* Paper presented at the World Association for Sexual Health conference, Sydney, Australia. Retrieved from https://tracieokeefe.com/autogynephilia-and-autoandrophilia-in-non-sex-and-gender-dysphoric-persons/

Olson K. R., Durwood, L., DeMeules, M. & McLaughlin,

Katie A. (2016). Mental health of transgender children who are supported in their identities. *Pediatrics*, 137(3).

Ramet, S. P. (1996). *Gender reversal & gender cultures.* Routledge.

Strauss, P., Cook, A., Winter, S., Watson, V., Wright Toussaint, D. & Lin, A. (2017). *Trans pathways: the mental health experiences and care pathways of trans young people.* Summary of results. Perth, Australia: Telethon Kids Institute.

Toomey R.B., Syvertsen A.K. & Shramko M. (2018). Transgender adolescent suicide behavior. *Pediatrics*, 142(4). doi: 10.1542/peds.2017-4218

Virupaksha, H., Muralidhar, D. & Ramakrishna, J. (2016). Suicide and suicidal behavior among transgender persons. *Indian Journal of Psychological Medicine*. doi: 10.4103/0253-7176.194908.

World Health Organization (2019), *Suicide: keys facts.* Retrieved from https://www.who.int/news-room/fact-sheets/detail/suicide

Zeluf, G., Dhejne, C., Orre, C., Mannheimer, L. N., Deogan, C., Höijer, J. Winzer, R. & Thorson, A.E. (2018). Targeted victimization and suicidality among trans people: A web-based survey. *LGBT Health*, 5(3). Retrieved from https://www.liebertpub.com/doi/10.1089/lgbt.2017.0011

Chapter 5:
The Effects of Discrimination

Discrimination happens in many ways but always has a profound detrimental effect on the people who experience it physically, psychologically, emotionally, socially and economically. All people from SGD groups experience discrimination in some form throughout their lives, regardless of any social privilege they may enjoy. Here we will discuss a few effects that discrimination can have on the lives of people from SGD groups.

Social psychology examines crowd mentality, conformity and how the average behaviour or manifested gestalt becomes the norm expected within groups and societies. In experiments, males tend to conform more than females (Carter et al., 2019) for fear of appearing female in any way, which explains why many men can be so aggressive and violent towards SGD groups. Coming from a SGD group will likely never be the norm, so their status will always be on the margins of society and subjected to discrimination, whether protected by anti-discrimination laws or not.

The establishment of male and female as the norm is in itself discrimination because many people straddle the area in-between sex and gender stereotypes. This area in-between is beginning to be more recognised as countries in many parts of the world change their laws to accommodate this population. However, at the time of writing, there is also a backlash in many places.

Before looking at some of the effects of discrimination, first let us first look at how research, academia and clinical practice has misinterpreted the suicidal drive in SGD groups. A typical example is the long-term follow-up study in Sweden of patients who went through sex reassignment treatment from 1973 to 2003 (Dhejne et al., 2011).

In the study, 324 sex-reassigned persons—191 male-to-females and 133 female-to-males—were matched against controls from the general population who were born in the same year of birth, and same natal-registered sex or destination sex. Results showed that post-transition patients were far more likely to have elevated psychiatric pathology, attempt and complete suicide than the control group. It was noted that reassignment for many, while perhaps alleviating a level of gender dysphoria, did not suffice as a treatment for transsexualism. It recommended that improved psychiatric and somatic care after sex reassignment should be provided for this patient group.

What the study completely missed was the level of social aggression from the public towards trans people in Sweden over those years. Also, the medical system that facilitated transition was highly misogynistic, authoritarian, oppressive and frequently patient-unfriendly. The legal system further failed to provide a wide range of sex and gender options other than a regimented male or female model. This forced many people with sex and gender issues into identities that were prescriptively male or female and not the destination that would have best accommodated some of those people's well-being. The very suggestion that people post-transition were psychiatrically dysfunctional was, in my view, transphobic discrimination and completely missed the social pressures that cause SGD minority stress.

We can see the rise of the extreme right-wing in America under the Trump administration, which sought to ban trans people with sex and gender differences from serving in the military (Dosh, 2019). A general sense of hopelessness, frustration and depression around the issue spread throughout the

American trans community when the Supreme Court initially upheld this ban that was enacted with no study or consultation with stakeholders. Soldiers from SGD groups who fought in combat for the US were suddenly no longer desirable. Even though they were fully functional as military personnel, they were made to feel disrespected by their Commander in Chief.

The policy on intersex people serving in the military was less clear (Marom et al., 2008). Intersex variations are profuse and often unclassifiable as many intersex people experience physiological anomalies in ways that no other person does. Further, many intersex people do not know they are intersex, and unless genetic tests or CT scans are carried out, neither would the doctors who examine them as they may appear to be fully functioning stereotypical males or females. Not everyone who is intersex has obvious characteristics. The military does not carry out such extensive physical examinations when personnel join the military or during their time of service.

So, we arrive at a situation where trans people may not serve in the US military but intersex people can as long as no-one knows they are intersex. Even if you are discovered to be intersex, you may have a similar body to a trans person but you may be allowed to continue to serve. Here we move into eugenics and body fascism.

For many professional trans soldiers who built their lives around the military, had families, mortgages and had served their country, serving a president who discriminated against them left them suffering minority stress. It pushed trans US military people back into the "don't ask, don't tell" policy era. Not only will many suffer combat fatigue and post-service depression, this situation, regardless of its reversal by President Biden, could raise the chances of suicidal ideation later in life due to post-traumatic minority stress.

We also see intersex groups discriminated against in medicine. Councillor Tony Biffa, an intersex man, accused

Melbourne Royal Children's Hospital (RCH), in Australia, of carrying out unnecessary surgeries on intersex children (Ferri, 2019). He demanded they withdraw from the Melbourne LGBTIQ+ Pride March because of their practices of abusing intersex children.

Biffa noted that local health services were provided for trans children who wanted to begin transition at puberty by taking hormone blockers to arrest puberty, which was a voluntary self-selected process carried out with the consent of the child. Yet, he argued, intersex children's reproductive surgeries were being carried out on them, when there was no biological need, without the person's permission, erasing their intersex status.

Biffa explained that removal and alteration of these tissues at such an early age, without their permission, does not take into account that they may feel violated later, as he did; it may also reduce their ability to enjoy sex. It is essentially forced so-called "normalisation" of intersex children based around shaming principles about the way they were born, instead of allowing them to make their own decision about what they want later in life. Many of these children do suffer depression and suicidal ideation around what was done to them later in life.

High-profile celebrities, such as multi-millionaire author of the *Harry Potter* books J.K. Rowling, have begun to express their views on SGD issues.

After expressing her support for "gender critical" feminists on Twitter, Rowling followed up with a blog post on her website (Rowling, 2020) to express her concern about what she sees as the erosion of women's sex-based rights. While acknowledging that she wants trans women to feel safe, Rowling says she does not want "natal" girls to feel unsafe by throwing open "the doors of bathrooms and changing rooms to any man who believes or feels he's a woman".

This kind of fear-mongering contributes to making people from SGD groups feel nervous, unsafe and oppressed, which can lead to depression and suicidal thoughts. Online comments particularly affect younger people who may be more connected and dependent on electronic communication as a large part of their social world.

"Cis privilege" according to Serano (2016) is the privilege enjoyed by people whose body and life trajectory is and has been heteronormative typical male and female, physically and socially. What people from SGD groups say is that heteronormative people do not know or are often unaware that they enjoy that privilege, just as many white middle-class Americans do not understand that they have privilege over poorer African Americans. When you act with disregard of your privilege in relationship to others, you are acting in a discriminatory way.

Frequently, cis privilege is a major problem for SGD groups because it can operate like a silent cancer without the perpetrators ever knowing or understanding they are being discriminatory. When people from SGD groups raise the issue of cis privilege, they are usually faced with amazement, incredulity and denial about what is happening.

It operates with attacks on people of sex and gender difference from certain radical feminists such as Germaine Greer (2014), Julie Bindel (Bell, 2016), Janice Raymond (1994), Cathy Brennan (Kohner, 2015) and Sheila Jeffreys (Bindel, 2005) who publicly verbally attack trans women and youth. Some of them may attempt to ban trans people from conferences, public events or sometimes contact the places where people work to malign them to their colleagues.

Intersex people get caught up in this discrimination because these radical feminists tend to display a lack of understanding about the diversity of biology and know very little about being intersex. They each enjoy cis privilege and seek to exclude trans women and thereby a number of intersex women from female spaces. It is othering and a denial of many women's rights.

Religious Discrimination

Religious persecution of people from SGD groups is such a large area that it could take up several volumes in itself. When religion becomes doctrine and departs from egalitarian humanistic philosophy, it evolves as chapter and verse dictatorialism, generally dominated by extreme misogyny that not only persecutes SGD groups but also women en masse.

Regardless of which Pope sits, the Catholic church constantly attacks SGD groups in the name of exclusivity in defence of the Adam and Eve creationist model of human nature. Women cannot be priests or hold positions of power in the church for fear that they may destabilise society with their presumed weakness and natural hysteria. Yet the church is largely supported by women's efforts within society to bind the family unit.

Historically many convents took in and protected intersex people along with others who did not fit in society. The Vatican castrated choir boys for hundreds of years until as late as 1959 so they could sing castrati with higher voices (Carroll, 2001). In 2019, in a papal document, Pope Francis heavily criticised modern gender theory and the very idea that gender was a matter of performance. He claimed it was an attempt to "annihilate the concept of nature". He further stated, "Efforts to go beyond the constitutive male-female sexual difference, such as the ideas of 'intersex' or 'transgender,' lead to a masculinity or femininity that is ambiguous" (McElwee, 2019).

While many ordinary Catholics may have a more humanitarian point of view, Catholic education takes a large part of its philosophy and guidance from the Vatican. This leads to children and adults subjected to a Catholic education being conflicted when they come from SGD groups, suffering profound guilt, shame, depression and suicidal thoughts. They may live a large part of their lives not claiming their real identity and hiding who and what they are from others for fear of rejection.

More liberal churches like the Church of England are only marginally more accepting of SGD groups. The Queen, who is the head of the Church, has always publicly embraced SGD groups, having them as guests in her homes, giving them awards and congratulating them on their social justice work. The late Queen Mother Elizabeth, Prince Charles and Prince William have behaved in the same way. The synod of the church, however, made up of highly conservative men, has publicly been homophobic, transphobic and intersexphobic, frequently leading to philosophical splits and divisions in the church (Sherwood, 2013).

In 2018, however, the Church of England's pastoral guidance to clergy and congregations stated, "The Church of England welcomes and encourages the unconditional affirmation of trans people, equally with all people, within the body of Christ, and rejoices in the diversity of that body into which all Christians have been baptised by one Spirit" (The Church of England, 2018). It specifically instructed that trans people and thereby all SGD Groups be addressed by any newly-declared names and identities.

While this may have been a move to welcome back those who had undergone full sex realignment treatment initially, by default it also included all SGD people and was a move to modernise the church in a time of dwindling attendances. It does, however, send strong messages of welcome and condemnation of discrimination that reverberates throughout the Churches of Scotland, Wales, Ireland and the rest of the protestant world. Congregants can be unafraid of people being from SGD groups, giving those groups an opportunity for better mental and physical health.

Mixed messages come from the Muslim faith in various countries such as Iran's teachings that to change your sex is acceptable (Why Iran is a Hub for Sex-Reassignment Surgery, 2019), but being homosexual means that society can put you to death (Weinthal, 2019). Back in the 1980s, Ayatollah Khomeini issued a fatwa that decreed 'sex changes' were acceptable and this has been supported by the current leaders.

Unfortunately, this pushes some gay people to change their gender rather than be put to death (Hamedani, 2014). Gay people in Iran experience an enormous amount of pressure from families, doctors, psychologists and the public to take hormones, have surgery and get their documents changed to the opposite sex, even under the threat of the family killing them for bringing shame on the family for being gay. Many later realised it was not the right move for them, suffered profound disenfranchisement in society and became depressed and suicidal.

In Malaysia, which is mainly a Muslim country, Religious Affairs Minister Zulkifli Mohamad declared in a Facebook post that he would give a "full license to all… enforcers" of the Federal Territories Islamic Religious Department to take action against transgender people in order to encourage them to "return to the right path" (Ewe, 2020). He was accused of inciting and legitimising state violence against trans people. Previously a mufti, Islamic jurist, he was once considered a friend of trans groups of people, having said, "As long as they do not use their identity for immoral purposes, it is not a shame and they are accepted in Islam".

Again, this is a country where gay sex is forbidden under Islamic law and criminalised under secular law in a male-led society. It is no stretch of the imagination to see that misogyny and homophobia reverberate into transhobia and intersexphobia. Only 14% of parliamentarians in Malaysia were women in 2019 and there were no openly trans or intersex people (Statistics, 2020). The adherence to strictly male and female stereotypes victimises those who are not achieving fully masculine or feminine social roles, citing them as moral dissidents.

Transgender women are known as "mak nyah", a non-stigmatising term. The words "transvestite" or "transsexual" can be used on government documents and reports (Human Rights Watch, 2014). Here we have a common situation where governments and the public often cannot distinguish between sex, gender and sexuality. What this means is that SGD groups get stigmatised by religious condemnation of sexualities that are other than heteronormative.

In 2014, a report titled *"I'm Scared to be a Woman"* (Human Rights Watch, 2014) noted how many trans women in Malaysia were constantly arrested, abused, beaten, put into prison and even blackmailed by the police for wearing women's clothing. A lot of the country practises sharia law, which frequently allows the police to be unaccountable because they are enforcing so-called religious morality. Consequently, trans people are framed by politicians as being non-Islamic.

Hinduism in general does not consider people who are from SGD groups as wholly male or female. Sexuality is rarely discussed in Hindu society but old temples may have carvings of sex between men and men and women and women, which was considered a sex education tool. It was only in 2018 that the Supreme Court of India decriminalised homosexuality, overturning attitudes left behind by the British colonisation that remained long after India became independent (Supreme Court Decriminalises Section 377, 2018; What is Section 377, 2020).

Again, before the British arrived en masse in India in the mid-19th century, many SGD people had a place in society. The displacement of culture by colonisation can never be underestimated and invading forces imprinted their sexual prejudices on those countries for generations. Hinduism has deities that have fluid genders as there are depictions of Shiva as an androgynous form with his wife, Parvati. The god Vishnu can appear as his female avatar Mohini. Gods can change gender legitimately within the faith and teachings (Davis, 2012).

SGD groups, however, suffer from discrimination in countries with large Hindu populations, not simply because of cultural displacement by colonisation, but also due to the caste or class systems. When you are a marginalised group and live in poverty due to that marginalisation, you become a victim of public disdain and disregard, leading to high levels of minority stress.

Buddhism, the fourth-biggest religion in the world, is less focused on persecution of any sector of society and is therefore more accepting of people from SGD groups (Human Rights Watch, n.d.). Some of its major tenets are not to do harm to others, refrain from killing or committing violence towards living beings and treating all beings with compassion and loving kindness. Teachings-wise, there are few references to sex, gender or sexuality diversity except that monks should refrain from intimate contact with others in order to preserve their spiritual focus, purpose and dedication.

While the Dali Lama once commented that "from a Buddhist point of view lesbian and gay sex is generally considered sexual misconduct", Buddhism in general considers opinions on sex and gender diversity as being a person's choice rather than having to fully rely on doctrine, of which there is little on this subject. This is not to say that SGD groups have an easier time in mainly Buddhist countries because there is often a lack of legislation that protects them against discrimination in places like Cambodia or Thailand (Fallon, 2020).

Regardless of where we may live, much of our lives and society are influenced by religious and societal belief systems that both consciously and unconsciously shape the structure of our personality and sub-personalities. These inform the way we see ourselves, others in relation to ourselves and the structure of our worldview, which can appear equitable or hostile and possibly traumatising and frightening.

People from SGD groups can be continually exposed to hostility throughout their lives due to the discriminatory influences of religion-based attitudes that pervade our societies. We as clinicians are constantly unaware consciously of the weight of those influences, frequently negative, upon the psyche of SGD clients that may lead them to depression, anxiety, trauma and suicide.

Therefore, we must always be sociologists in executing our duties so we can filter out the unseen cultural variables that drove the client to the edge of a death wish. At times, we may even have to engage with the client in cultural or religious deprogramming, belief evolution and re-education to take them away from those prejudicial, falsely-constructed discriminatory beliefs about their lack of value.

Public Discrimination in Entertainment and the Media

Public scorn and debasement are a common everyday experience for many people from SGD groups. When you do not look like the average person, you stand out in the crowd. When people want someone to attack, those who stand out become easy targets for the anger and psychopathy of others.

In 2014, the American television personality Clayton Morris had to apologise for comments that he made on air while appearing on a Valentine's Day segment of *Fox & Friends* (Frazier, 2014). When discussing Facebook's new gender options, he jokingly told co-host Elisabeth Hasselbeck that he had changed his gender on Facebook to "intersex". It was clear he did not know what intersex was, could not distinguish between sex and gender and thought it was a joke, causing many intersex people to be offended by his comments. For intersex people struggling to have their issues taken seriously, they felt him referring to their sex issues as gender issues was disempowering.

During the COVID-19 crisis, Dr Rachel Levine, a trans woman, was subjected to a cascade of mockery and abuse on social media and elsewhere (Rubinkam, 2020). As Pennsylvania's Health Secretary, she had to give television appearances regarding the handling of the statewide response to the coronavirus pandemic. There were comments like "a man in a dress" and many more abusive public comments. The public comments were nothing to do with her professional performance during the crisis but simply an onslaught of transphobia.

Marvel Comics came under severe criticism when unveiling its plans for a new non-binary superhero called "Snowflake" (Hitch, 2020). While the creators of the character were a cisgendered man and a queer artist attempting to be at the cutting-edge of storytelling, they seemed unaware of wider non-binary politics. The term "snowflake" is an insult and denotes someone who is delicate, irrational, weak and neurotic, giving the reader the impression that underneath the superhero's status there are endemic character flaws. This made non-binary people angry because to be non-binary in society actually takes a great deal of strength and the act of naming the character "Snowflake" was considered insulting. They felt that the storytelling would give the wrong messages.

Public debasement, particularly when it is constant, eats away at a person's sense of self-worth and confidence, at times to the extent that people lose the will to live. When that debasement is founded on discrimination against a person, as not all people are strong or superheroes, they can experience a sense of powerlessness and hopelessness. The victim can begin to believe the derogatory comments and bullying, seeing themselves as wrong and at fault.

When the discrimination is directly or aimlessly targeted at SGD groups, it runs the danger of escaping critique under the guise of entertainment. There is little doubt that SGD groups are some of the most disadvantaged groups in the world today who are constantly campaigning for the recognition of their human rights. Such progress and community sense of well-being, however, can be severely damaged by a general gestalt of insults and public mockery. As clinicians working with SGD groups, to be authentic, we have no other choice but to be political in the way we carry out our duties and challenge the harm caused by discrimination and bullying at every turn.

Per capita, people known to be from SGD groups also tend to have lower socioeconomic prospects when they are deselected in work situations, forced into poverty and then suffer mental health and somatic issues due to that poverty (Mani, 2013; National Center on Transgender Equality, 2015; Jones et al., 2016). The presupposition that people have extreme mental health issues simply because they are from SGD groups is endemic throughout medicine, society and the law.

So, when a person from a SGD group presents themselves, they can immediately encounter a wall of superstitions based on prejudice, negative misconceptions and falsely-based generalisations. Covert discrimination is much subtler but nonetheless just as prevalent as overt discrimination. It operates by deselection from opportunities, appropriation of narrative and blanking out of SGD groups' existence in the public arena.

It happens behind closed doors but also on the public stage by not inviting SGD groups to represent themselves. If we consider that the percentage of people from SGD groups seen publicly in our society is around a 1–2%-plus variant, it is curious to see a general scarcity of representation from those groups in medicine, entertainment, politics, academia, economics, journalism, law, and society in general.

Covert discrimination has also been big in the gay/queer/ LGBTI culture as appropriation of SGD narratives takes place when lesbian and gay people attempt to speak on behalf of people from SGD groups but do not invite them to speak for themselves. In other words, it is infantilisation and the erasure of SGD people's intelligence, presence and the importance of their own SGD voices. Individuals and groups are left feeling unheard, discounted, ignored and mostly disrespected. If you do not have a voice, how can you discuss your issues, fears and value? How can you ask for what you need to stay alive with quality of life, avoid despair and choose an alternative to suicide?

Discrimination extends to misrepresentation in the press, which frequently misgenders people in order to create clickbait. The *Samoa Observer* was heavily criticised for unethical reporting and publishing a photo of the dead body of Jeanine Tuivaiki on their front page following her suicide. She was faafafine but the reporter constantly referred to her as "he" (Tapaleao, 2016). The Prime Minster of Samoa, Mr Malielegaoi, said, "As a parent, it was devastating to see someone's child portrayed in such a heartless manner." He also acknowledged that the actions of *The Observer* were clearly against the country's cultural beliefs. Not only is the individual disrespected by being misrepresented in the media in this way, but so are their family and community.

The British trans lobbying group Press for Change, which campaigns for trans people's rights, was started in the early 1990s partly as a reaction to misrepresentation in the media. Its efforts to gain legal recognition for trans people was constantly supported with the effort to create better representation in the media. Professor Stephen Whittle has spoken about how British trans people had lived in the shadows trying to be unobserved until the 1990s. Generally, when they appeared in the media it was mostly in a sensationalist story written by tabloid journalists trying to get a headline so this was how the public saw trans people: in a negative light (Trans Activist Stephen Whittle on Facing Abuse On TV, 2018).

The BBC attacked trans charities by dropping The Gender Trust, Mermaids and The Gender Identity Research and Education Society (GIRES) from their Action Line website (Parson, 2020). These organisations had provided decades of support and advice to the community. In an email from BBC Pride, they said, "It is a complex area and the BBC needs to remain impartial". In reality, they caved to complaints from right-wing bigotry that claim the charities harm children when in fact they have helped save the lives of thousands of children over the years.

A spokesperson for the charity Mermaids commented saying, "This happened at a time of growing transphobia in wider society". Since the BBC is considered a worldwide source of reliable information, even though it has previously shown few representations of SGD groups, it now gives the impression that being from an SGD group is somehow improper, wrong and offensive. This is a prime example of right-wing politics and crowd victimisation invading mass media outlets and enacting institutionalised discrimination. Imagine for one moment the outcry if the BBC had removed charities for the blind, deaf or aged.

Social and Economic Discrimination
One of the most common effects of discrimination is social and economic exclusion and sometimes by sectors one might initially think would be supportive of SGD groups (Hoffman, 2020). In July 2020, Barbados passed laws to protect gay and lesbian people against discrimination, particularly in the workplace. LGBT organisations did not call out the government and politicians when they failed to include trans people in the bill. Frequently, trans was labelled as being a sexual orientation, not a sex or gender identity. Rather than endangering the bill by pushing for sex and gender identity to be included, gay campaigners let the exclusion ride.

Alexa Hoffman, a trans woman who had been suspended from her job in a legal firm for changing her name and daring to stand up as trans, commented, "Much like my case, if a trans person is prejudiced out of their job, they will be forced to undertake extensive and expensive legal research to get justice. And many employers will continue to discriminate against us because they assume that we will not be in a position to seek redress."

This kind of institutionalised discrimination can be very oppressive to people from SGD groups as it suggests a sense of legitimate approval of such discrimination and appears to confirm the notion that SGD groups are somehow wrong. Such views can become contagious and spread like an uncontrollable wildfire, misleading the public.

When people from SGD groups find themselves marginalised by other minorities and sidelined by gay issues, it is a hard blow psychologically and emotionally, leaving some with a sense of hopelessness, despondency and depression. People from SGD groups are frequently excluded from intersectionality because their issues are seen as too complex to understand or politically manoeuvre. That constant erasure or threat of erasure leads many to live on a knife-edge of chronic fear.

It is clear from a review of published papers, studies and analysis, sourced from different countries, that SGD groups of people can experience high levels of suicidal thoughts, attempts and successful suicides, far in excess of the general populous. They are always minority groups in any culture and those groups can be vulnerable to rejection by families, employment, society or religious movements, causing low levels of self-worth, hopelessness and a sense of oppression, which clearly increases the risk of suicide.

While studies often conflate the identities of these subpopulations, colouring them with attributes they do not possess, it is useful from an academic and sociological perspective to consider them as simply SGD groups of people. What is clear from the results is that many of the stress factors that create suicidal ideation and lead to suicide attempts and successful suicide overlap between the different groups.

These stressors include forced medical treatment, lack of access to medical treatment, poverty and inability to afford medical treatment, the stress of dealing with chronic health conditions related to sex and/or gender, mistreatment by healthcare professionals, being missexed and misgendered, stigma, lack of acceptance of their sex and/or gender identity, bullying at school and in the workplace, deselection from work and study opportunities, social isolation and enforced poverty, lack of legal protection against discrimination, inability to gain legal documents that support their sex and gender status, marginalisation, difficulties maintaining personal relationships, rejection by families and their religion, homelessness, harassment, threats of violence, violence and assault, failure of police protection and respectful treatment, lack of positive reinforcement around their sex and/or gender experiences, at times regret at changing their body and gender identity, drug and alcohol addiction to deal with the stressors, a sense of hopelessness, depression, fear, being unsafe in the world, post-traumatic stress disorder due to harassment, the constant threat that right-wing politicians will attempt to take away their civil rights and a sense of foreboding that leads to increased mental health issues.

As noted in previous chapters, all of these can contribute to up to ten times and above the national suicide risk in a wide range of countries, even ones that have national anti-discrimination laws.

The rejection and discrimination SGD groups of people experience can lead to marginalisation, fear, depression, neurosis, mental health complications and a sense of being unsafe in the world. This reduces their quality of life and ostracises them from mainstream culture with reduced life opportunities. The ensuing fear for their safety and sense of danger can lead to suicidal thoughts, self-harm, low self-esteem and in many cases successful suicide.

In an egalitarian and democratic society, the United Nations Charter of Human Rights leads us to believe that all citizens should be treated equally before the law and in society regardless of identity, disability or difference. It is clear from the research reviewed that this is not the case for people who come from many SGD groups. Not only are they frequently treated in a demeaning, harmful and debilitating manner, many of them also believe that life is too perilous and extremely limited for them, which can lead to suicidal thoughts.

What, above all, is most notable about the research reviewed are the clear correlations between SGD groups' sense of rejection, isolation, bullying and abandonment by families, discrimination from educational institutions, healthcare providers, peers and society in general. Combine those with people's experiences and we can see high levels of mental health issues, inflating the risk of suicidal ideation and attempts.

In recent years, medical, psychological and social models have been transitioning from a disease-based model of people from SGD groups to a health-based model. This change in attitude has mainly come about due to the actions of social justice and advocacy movements that have lobbied for depathologisation of these populations.

This, however, has not been and is not a smooth pathway of acceptability within the public arena. It is constantly assaulted by religious extremists who use SGD groups as political footballs and subject them to public attacks from medical professionals who are unable to accept the reality of the diversity of sex and gender. These attacks and social rejections of people from SGD groups adds to their fear for personal safety, anxiety, depression, trauma, and reduces quality of life. This in turn elevates the levels of minority stress on an individual and group basis, leading towards higher suicide ideations, attempted and successful suicides, and creating highly vulnerable populations.

While suicidality is often viewed as a psychopathology and a disturbance of the balance of the mind for SGD groups, it appears in general to be a reaction to a sense of extreme minority stress and hopeless. In SGD populations, it is clear that suicidal drivers are not solely based on an existential crisis of being or feeling unable to cope, but are frequently triggered by post-traumatic stress and a fear for safety, harm to dignity, and a sense of extreme long-term or sudden onset doom-laden thinking for an individual in what, at times, seems to be an insurmountable personal situation.

Sports writer Mike Penner of the *Los Angeles Times*, considered a first-rate journalist, died at 52 in 2009 of suicide. A gifted writer, he transitioned and lived as Christine Daniels in 2007 and was honoured at the National Gay and Lesbian Journalists Association at its convention in San Diego for telling her story. In her first column discussing transition, Penner (2007) came out and wrote, "I am a transsexual sports writer. It has taken more than 40 years, a million tears and hundreds of hours of soul-wrenching therapy for me to work up the courage to type those words."

Confused and struggling with their identity, they transitioned back in 2008 and, according to a friend, seemed to find life too difficult, embarrassed about their double transition and unable to discuss it with people (Thursby, 2009). Regardless of how much therapy people may have undergone, for some people, struggling with sex and gender issues can be too overwhelming, leading them to suicide.

In Chennai, India, a 19-year-old transsexual woman identified as Sabina abandoned her two-wheeler on the side of the road after noticing the police patrolling at Valluvar Kottam junction (Chennai: 19-Year-Old Transsexual Hangs Self to Death, 2020). The police seized the unattended vehicle and took it to the police station. When Sabina went to the police station to try and collect it, the police told her to bring her documents. Upset that she had to produce identity documents, which can often not be coordinated with how a person may now be living, she hanged herself. It is very hard for many

SGD groups to gain official documents that match their chosen identities.

For some people, the excruciating pain and embarrassment of having to produce documents that disclose their birth registered status, which can open them up to discrimination, can be so overwhelming and daunting that they would prefer to die by suicide.

References

Bell, S. (2016). NUS 'right to have no platform policy'. *BBC News*. Retrieved from https://www.bbc.com/news/education-36101423

Bindel, J. (2005, July 2). The ugly side of beauty. *The Guardian*. Retrieved from www.theguardian.com/world/2005/jul/02/gender.politicsphilosophyandsociety

Carroll, T. (2001). Pope urged to apologise for Vatican castrations. *The Guardian*. Retrieved from https://www.theguardian.com/world/2001/aug/14/humanities.highereducation

Carter, M., Franz, T., Gruschow, J. & VanRyne, A. (2019). The gender conformity conundrum: The effects of irrelevant gender norms on public conformity. *The Journal of Social Psychology*, 159(6).

Chennai: 19-year-old transsexual hangs self to death after police seize her vehicle. (2020, July, 11). *Mirror Now Digital*. Retrieved from www.timesnownews.com/mirror-now/crime/article/chennai-19-year-old-transsexual-hangs-self-to-death-after-police-seize-her-vehicle/620035

Church of England. (2018). Guidance for welcoming transgender people published. Retrieved from www.churchofengland.org/more/media-centre/news/

guidance-welcoming-transgender-people-published

Davis, R. (2020). *Gods in print: Masterpieces of India's mythological art.* Mandala Publishing.

Dhejne, C., Lichtenstein P., Boman M., Johansson A.L.V., Långström N. & Landén M. (2011). Long-term follow-up of transsexual persons undergoing sex reassignment surgery: Cohort study in Sweden. *Plos One.* Retrieved from https://doi.org/10.1371/journal.pone.0016885

Dosh, R. (2019, June 24). I was discharged from the military for being trans. I'm losing hope of ever serving again. What the Supreme Court's latest decision on the trans military ban means. *Vox.* Retrieved from https://www.vox.com/first-person/2019/1/24/18195975/trump-trans-military-ban-supreme-court-decision

Ewe, K. (2020). Malaysian official grants 'full license' to arrest, 'educate' transgender people. *Vice.* Retrieved from https://www.vice.com/en_au/article/ep45dp/malaysian-official-grants-full-license-arrest-educate-transgender

Fallon, A. (2020). The shocking reality of life for transgender women in Cambodia, Fallon. *SBS.* Retrieved from https://www.sbs.com.au/topics/pride/agenda/article/2016/11/02/shocking-reality-life-transgender-women-cambodia

Ferri, L. (2019). Intersex councillor claims hospital is performing 'traumatising involuntary procedures on intersex children' which force them to be male or female. *Daily Mail Australia.* Retrieved from https://www.dailymail.co.uk/news/article-6626265/Intersex-Melbourne-councillor-claims-hospital-performing-involuntary-procedures-intersex-children.html

Frazier, A. (2014). Fox news anchor apologizes for 'ignorant' joke about gender identity. *Advocate*. Retrieved www. advocate.com/politics/media/2014/03/04/fox-news-anchor-apologizes-ignorant-joke-about-gender-identity

Greer, G. (2014). *The whole woman*. Transworld Digital.

Hamedani, A. (2014). The gay people pushed to change their gender. *BBC News*. Retrieved from www.bbc.com/news/ magazine-29832690

Hitch, M. (2020). Backlash as Marvel unveils first non-binary superhero. *Star Observer*. Retrieved from https://www. starobserver.com.au/news/backlash-as-marvel-unveils-first-non-binary-superhero/193827

Hoffmann, A. (2020, July 30). Barbados legislates anti-trans bigotry. *76 Crimes*. Retrieved from https://76crimes. com/2020/07/30/barbados-legislates-anti-trans-bigotry/

Human Rights Watch. (2014). Malaysia: Transgender people under threat. Retrieved from https://www.hrw.org/news /2014/09/24/malaysia-transgender-people-under-threat

Human Rights Watch. (n.d.). Stances of faiths on LGBTQ issues: Buddhism. Retrieved from https://www.hrc.org/ resources/stances-of-faiths-on-lgbt-issues-buddhism

Jones, T., Hart, B., Carpenter, M., Ansara, G., Leonard, W. & Lucke, J. (2016). Intersex: Stories and statistics from Australia. Retrieved from https://interactadvocates.org/ wp-content/uploads/2016/01/Intersex-Stories-Statistics-Australia.pdf

Kohner, C. (2015, January 25). Sorry about your dick: An interview with Cathy Brennan, Why Cathy Brennan blocked me on Twitter and Facebook. Planet Transgender. Retrieved from https://planettransgender.com/ sorry-about-your-dick-an-interview-with-cathy-brennan/

Mani; Joseph, D. (2013). Social exclusion of transgender: problems and prospects. *Indian Social Science Journal*. Retrieved from https://search.proquest.com/docview/1471982998

Marom, T., Itskoviz, D. & Ostfeld, I. (2008). Intersex patients in military service. *Military Medicine*, 173(11), 1132-1135. Retrieved from https://doi.org/10.7205/MILMED.173.11.1132

McElwee, J. (2019, June 10). Vatican office blasts gender theory, questions intentions of transgender people. *National Catholic Reporter*. Retrieved from https://www.ncronline.org/news/vatican/vatican-office-blasts-gender-theory-questions-intentions-transgender-people

National Center on Transgender Equality. (2015). Report from the National Center on Transgender Equality 2015 U.S. Transgender Survey. Retrieved from https://www.ustranssurvey.org/

Parsons, V. (2020), 'Disgraceful' BBC accused of 'bowing to deliberate hate' after quietly cutting ties with trans charities. *Pink News*. Retrieved from https://www.pinknews.co.uk/2020/07/30/bbc-pride-trans-hate-campaign-mermaids-action-line-transphobia-gender-trust/

Penner, M. (2007, April 26). Old Mike, new Christine. *Los Angeles Times*. Retrieved from https://www.latimes.com/sports/la-sp-oldmike26apr26-story.html

Raymond, J. (1994). *The transsexual empire: The making of the she-male* (Athene series). Teachers College Press.

Rowling, J.K. (2020). J.K. Rowling writes about her reasons for speaking out on sex and gender issues [Blog post]. Retrieved from https://www.jkrowling.com/opinions/j-k-rowling-writes-about-her-reasons-for-speaking-out-on-sex-and-gender-issues/

Rubinkam, M. (2020). Transgender official takes abuse while leading virus efforts. *ABC News*. Retrieved from https://abcnews.go.com/US/wireStory/transgender-official-takes-abuse-leading-virus-efforts-71902013

Serano, Julia. *Whipping girl: A transsexual woman on sexism and the scapegoating of femininity.* 2nd ed. Seal Press.

Sherwood, H. (2017, February 15). Church of England in turmoil as synod rejects report on same-sex relationships. *The Guardian*. Retrieved from https://www.theguardian.com/world/2017/feb/15/church-of-england-in-turmoil-as-synod-rejects-report-on-same-sex-relationships

Statistica. (2020). Proportion of seats held by women in national parliaments in Malaysia from 2005 to 2019. Retrieved from https://www.statista.com/statistics/730186/malaysia-proportion-of-seats-held-by-women-in-national-parliament/

Supreme Court decriminalises Section 377: All you need to know. (2018). *Times of India*. Retrieved from https://timesofindia.indiatimes.com/india/sc-verdict-on-section-377-all-you-need-to-know/articleshow/65695884.cms

Tapaleao, V. (2016, June 20). Samoan PM blasts newspaper over dead trans woman on front page. *NZ Herald*. Retrieved from https://www.nzherald.co.nz/nz/news/article.cfm?c_id=1&objectid=11659908

Thursby, K. (2009, November 29). Mike Penner dies at 52. Los Angeles Times sportswriter. *Los Angeles Times*. Retrieved from www.latimes.com/archives/la-xpm-2009-nov-29-la-me-mike-penner29-2009nov29-story

Trans activist Stephen Whittle on facing abuse on TV. (2018, May 29). *BBC News*. Retrieved from https://www.bbc.

com/news/av/education-44240899

What is section 377 of IPC? (2020). *Times of India.* Retrieved from https://timesofindia.indiatimes.com/india/what-is-section-377/articleshow/66067994.cms

Chapter 6:
Clinical Mistakes

Unquestionably bad clinical choices have been scattered throughout the treatment of sex and gender diverse (SGD) groups. This poor decision-making by professionals impacts the lives of patients for decades and sometimes life. Many of them have led the clients to a poor state of mental health in the short- or long-term and in many cases resulted in suicide. For a large part, this is unrecorded and mostly under-reported.

In the theory of social medicine, there are initially two diametrically-opposed schools around delivery of service. The first is the bourgeoisie approach, which is where the doctor knows best and is in charge (Cockerham, 2013). They are pitched as trained professionals and the patient needs to be subservient to their knowledge. If you have been in a car accident and had arteries severed, lying on a gurney in the emergency department, you are probably best to allow the medical staff to be in charge so they can save your life.

The opposite theory is an interactive egalitarian model of medicine where the approach is that the client and the clinician make decisions together. This can be useful when the outcome of any treatment cannot be reasonably guaranteed and may even be experimental, so the patient really does need to be held responsible for the outcome as much as the clinician.

There is a third competing theory, but it is not so prevalent in Western medicine and that is when the community makes the medical decisions. This often happens in native, Indigenous cultures when the community together listens to the stories, considers the options and spends time talking about the situation to reach a decision.

Surgery

Modern surgical sex affirmation treatments have been for around 150 years in medicine although thousands of years ago males would drink the urine of pregnant mares to feminise as well as undergo castration. The fact that castration was used until the 1950s by the Catholic church to raise the pitch of the voices of male sopranos conveniently escapes the condemnation of the Vatican. *The Bible* actually refers to born and made eunuchs (New International Version, 1973/2011, Matthew 19).

Early surgeries to correct genital anomalies were being experimented with in the late part of the 19th century. The introduction of anaesthesia allowed surgeons to perform more radical surgeries without the patient experiencing such high levels of body shock. Hijra, however, have practised penile amputation for centuries, often crudely and sometimes creating infection, in their desperation to be demasculinised.

The creation of neo-vaginas or removal of a hypertrophic clitoris in intersex people who are born without vaginas or have developmental differences has become standard practice in surgery. The creation of neo-vaginas in trans women has developed from crude castration and amputation of the penis to higher levels of pelvic surgery that allows surgeons to create cosmetically functioning vaginas for penetrative sex. Also, external fashioning of labia, clitoral and urethral tissue has been able to produce, in many cases, sensate, functioning female genitalia.

Repair and creation of male genitalia have developed considerably over the last 40 years, particularly with the advancement of using different donor sites for skin and tissue harvesting. The introduction of phalloplasty, metoidioplasty and genital prosthesis has also aided surgeons to create more aesthetically authentic and functioning male genitalia.

The introduction of facial feminisation surgery, breast construction and chest sculpting has further advanced cosmetic and functional sex differentiation procedures. What was once experimental cosmetic surgery has now become more mainstream. However, a surgeon can only work with the material that is before them so they must carry out the surgery with the tissue they have; sometimes patients can have too high an expectation of what may be done for them and can be disappointed by the results.

Advertising and patient reports also now play a large role in surgical consumerism. What may look like a marvellous outcome on the internet may not be possible for everyone. Some surgeons do not always tell patients of the dangers and risks of surgery even though all patients sign disclaimer forms before surgery to exonerate the surgeon from mishaps; in truth, few patients ever read those forms before signing them.

Surgery is an art as well as a science. A surgeon learns by their mistakes as well as their successes, like any craftsperson. Unfortunately, a lot of sex differentiation surgery over the years has been offered by surgeons who do not have the experience or talent and have produced poor results and disasters that severely affect the patient's mental health; this can, at times, result in the patient considering or completing suicide.

With intersex people and people with non-stereotypical sex characteristics, the delivery of service has for so long taken the bourgeoisie approach where the doctors always know best. Doctors have foisted and forced surgeries on children to try to make their genitals look typically male or female.

Some of those surgeries can produce an inability to enjoy sex and a failure of the sex response when tissue, including nerves, is removed. Incontinence and scarring may also occur. The excuse of trying to make the child appear "normal", driven by the theory that they will grow up psychologically balanced, is not proven, and many people who experienced that surgery testify to the opposite, in that it permanently psychologically damaged their life.

Hiding those childhood medical records from these people as adults is also damaging. Some people have spent decades trying to find out what has actually medically been done to them and how that affected them. They may understand that the clinician was trying to do what they thought was best for the patient. In reality, however, it was not the clinician's right to make those decisions and was basically a medical assault upon the child, justified by the exaltation of supposed correct "normality".

Parents were frequently vulnerable, having felt over-whelmingly pressured to allow those procedures by doctors and medical staff who convinced them the child will be "normal" afterwards. They were told that other children would surely bully their child if such procedures were not performed or the child would be maladjusted physically and mentally.

Even though it may have not been a medical emergency, the child being intersex was treated as an affront to human-ity with the presumption that their intersex diversity should always be corrected and erased. It was framed as a biological mistake that the child carries with them for life as they are deemed to have begun life as and remained wrong. Those med-ics can convince the parents that it is a decision that should never be left to the child when they become older because that would be too late to fix the supposed wrongness.

There is also the issue of health services not providing sufficient services for intersex children and adults who need medical intervention. Budgets are often not allocated for these services or they are downgraded against other services as being non-essential. Clinicians may have to itemise the procedures in the state medical system or private health insurance under other procedures to provide the patient with the care they need. This puts intersex people in a very precarious stressful position.

The mistakes of those doctors, healthcare practitioners, governments, politicians and social influencers wishing to eradicate the conversation around non-medical emergency surgery denies intersex validity. We can see in Utah the comments by Merrill Nelson, a Republican politician, on the proposed Bill 153 into state parliament to ban any change of markers on birth certificates (Hinkle, 2019). Nelson said he did not believe the bill was driven by hate or phobia, but he works for a law firm that represents the Mormon Church, which touts creationism and is critical of sex and/or gender diversity. This persistent opposition to intersex existence leads to depression in many intersex people who live in fear about the reintroduction of laws that erase their existence.

What is important to note here is that the patient's opinions have generally been ignored and while some interventions have provided satisfactory results for the patient, many have left people very unhappy with the results. Hence now we have the intersex movement that is calling for all non-medical emergency intervention to be suspended until a person or child is fully informed of their options so they can decide for themselves.

The intersex movement believes that early, non-consensual intervention is clearly and equivocally an assault. Some doctors are complying while others are protesting that they know best without producing sufficient follow-up data of patient satisfaction. The sheer number of these non-consensual surgery cases have been hidden from the public and not been reported in the literature.

Many people from SGD groups, however, have benefited massively from various surgeries. In such cases, it has been successful and it has clearly saved their lives and brought them back from suicide. To live with a body that is physically not functioning or not in line with how a person perceives themselves to be is a burden. When surgery can resolve that sense of dysphoria, we have a duty as health professionals to guide clients in that direction but always with their consent.

Therapy

Patients desperate for remedies for the physical, mental and social problems associated with sex and gender dysphoria are drawn at times to what seems like a solution but occasionally turns out not to be the nirvana they sought. Surgeries do go wrong and patients do make mistakes about what they may be seeking in their lives, sometimes blaming the clinicians and trying to sue them.

Psychological and psychotherapeutic screening and care before irreversible procedures is wise and any surgeon would be wise to require it before they operate. If you are going to move to another continent, it is wise to take advice before you pack up your belongings and wave goodbye. If you change professions, you need to train in the new profession and be prepared to do the work it takes to become skilled in that new profession.

Many people who struggle with their sex and gender issues, however, do not think they need to do that work. They become hostile at the very suggestion they should do the psychological work in therapy to adjust to their situation and insist they are making the right decisions. They may say it is too expensive and they have the right to make their own decisions; but having a detached person reflect back to you your decisions and their consequences in a safe, respectful space is useful for people to gain clarity.

Where we have often run into trouble with the delivery of services to people from SGD groups is that the delivery of services has sometimes swung far too much towards bourgeoise medicine or permissive freedom of choice. Any curtailing of instant freedom of choice is considered abuse by many SGD human rights campaigners but a decision to change your body or your social gender presentation can lead to a life of regret and suicide when not considered carefully.

It can be highly stressful being intersex at times due to encountering high medical bills and dealing with social ostracisation or the push to conform to being strictly male or female. For some these medical bills can be a lifelong expense and daunting, and many families simply could not afford that care.

Counselling and psychotherapy are often not offered to intersex people to help them manage their lives. Clinics generally only offer physical treatment options, expecting clients to cope with the mental and emotional problems they may encounter from being intersex. This can often lead to depression and suicidal thoughts.

Also, the psychoanalytical field espoused the concept that someone who did not want to appear male or female did so because of some kind of childhood trauma and the job of the psychoanalyst was to spend years digging into the patient's mind to find out the cause of the maladjustment. Even if people were intersex and they wanted to claim their true identity as intersex, they were considered maladjusted if they did not settle down to the sex that had been ascribed. Only the cases who were seen as hopeless were considered for transition but then the analysts still classified them as maladjusted. Only in 2019 did the American Psychoanalytic Association apologise for decades of mislabelling that surely drove some people from SGD groups to suicide (Murphy, 2019).

The problem with these top-down/top dog approaches to therapy is that the clinician decides what the patient should be and does their best to force them to conform to their diagnosis. The patient's opinions are not really important or relevant to the therapy. The problem that arises from this way of working is the clinicians get it wrong a great deal of the time because they ascribe rather than observe and listen. In this approach, clinicians put their theory before the observation, instead of the observation before the theory, which can cause high levels of distress and suicidal thoughts in SGD clients.

Psychiatry

Some of the greatest thinkers in psychiatry, like Laing (1964) and Szasz (2007), have challenged the fundamental concepts of persistent pathologisation and have instead taken a more humanistic approach to people's problem-solving. Those who have often taken that approach around SGD issues have frequently been hounded and harassed by the psychiatric establishment, which is essentially bourgeoise.

The attempt by psychiatry to possess and dominate the lives of SGD people by classifications in the American Psychiatric Association's *Diagnostic & Statistical Manual of Mental Disorders* (DSM) (APA, 1980) and the World Health Organization's (1988) *International Classification of Diseases* (ICD, 10) have failed. For many years, psychiatry tried to control the lives of people from SGD groups by attempting to cure them of a mental illness they did not have. Clinicians pushed people into unrealistic behavioural programs such as electric shock therapy or aversion therapy to assimilate them into being "normal" men or women.

Again, this was controlled by commercialised pathologisation and the strategy of instilling shame and wrongness. One of the highest criteria for a patient was that the public should not find out about a patient's history. If the public found out the patient was from a SGD group, they would have failed to become a "normal" person. People who went through transition clinics such as Johns Hopkins (USA) and Charing Cross Hospital (UK) were given the clear directive that the exercise aimed to make clients as normal as possible. If the client failed to pass as what the clinician regarded as "normal" in the street, they carried with them the burden of having been considered a clinical disaster.

If there were any doubts in the clinician's mind that someone could not pass in the street as a stereotypical male or female after transition, the patient could be dismissed from the care program. These clinics were generally run by authoritarian male tyrants who frequently gained professorships on the back of the abuse they were perpetrating.

Many of the people who were dismissed and turned away from those psychiatry- and psychology-controlled programs turned to drugs and alcohol to kill their emotional pain and large numbers of them completed suicide by one form or another. Being intersex in those programs gave you no advantage as you were judged solely on whether you could eventually pass as strictly male or female. That was the gold standard. In parts of the world today, this same philosophy is still practised.

In the 1970s, I used to visit trans women and men who were trying to get into the British National Health System's Charing Cross Hospital transition program, which I went through myself. Many were desperate, had no money for private care and could be suicidal. Some of the unrecorded souls that I had contact with, who passed through the brutal, authoritarian Charing Cross Hospital in the 1960s, 70s and early 80s, were Don, Ray, Sophie, Carmen, Carole, Stacy, Anna, Linda, Ena, Perl, Karen, Jade, Viviane and Mandy, to name a few, all of whom died of drugs or alcohol, some accidental and some intentional.

No kind of counselling or psychotherapy was available to them so their transition was stressful and they never learnt to deal with their new reality and survival living as women or men. Those patients were often treated at the hospital as if they were criminals. Many, rejected by families and society, ended up working in the sex industry for large parts of their lives. I had to visit many in secret for fear of being persecuted by the clinician for interfering with their patient.

The clinicians decided whether you were intersex, transsexual (later transgender), a supposed disaffected, confused cross-dresser or wasting their time with delusions of passing as male or female when they thought you could not. If you did not have the money to go privately, these government-run institutions in different countries had the monopoly on who would get help and who would not.

Another unrecorded soul was Maureen, a full-time cross-dresser who was harassed by the police for a large part of her life just for her very existence. She was always moving home in the UK, always going from one menial job to another to survive and avoid harassment. She was classified as a public pervert and a danger to society by the police.

There was also Sheila who lived in an abandoned warehouse by Shepherd's Bush roundabout in London. She was rejected for sex reassignment treatment at Charing Cross Hospital because the clinician believed she could not pass as a woman. Every day, she would walk to Soho in the West End to play her fiddle for coins. She was a gifted musician, but the public would spit on her as they passed in disdain. Eventually, she died of pneumonia in the middle of a freezing winter in an empty warehouse where she was squatting with no heating.

I could tell you similar stories of intersex and trans women and men I met when I lived in France, Italy, Spain, Holland, Greece and America. These amount to thousands of people abused by clinicians and they should be remembered. My colleagues in other countries could also tell you about an equal number of cases of clinical abuse and mistakes they came across.

The history of SGD people should never be buried. Neither should it be lilac-washed as our historians often only write tales of successful people when, in reality, the history of SGD people includes horrendous discrimination and mistreatment that led many people to suicide.

The same situation had been happening with hormonal intervention, masculinising and feminising people without fully informing them of what is happening and why, failing to keep proper medical records and hiding facts from patients. Later in life when patients discover the real facts, they can feel deceived, betrayed and abused, and want to change their bodies to other than the doctor thought it should become. The trauma of that discovery can lead to complex trauma and thoughts of suicide.

Withholding treatment when it is appropriate is clinical abuse. Withholding information and education around sex and/or gender diversity is also abuse. Whether it is withholding services in religious schools, higher education or medical settings, it is all abuse. As the movie star and ex-Governor of California Arnold Schwarzenegger said, "There are no two sides to hatred" (Washington, 2017). Neither children nor adults can make an informed decision unless they have the full scientific facts about themselves and their options, so they have a right to sufficient information about their choices.

The withholding of treatment or lack of funding around treatment for those who experience sex or gender dysphoria is clinical abuse. Some politicians and healthcare professionals may espouse that they know better about the situation than the patient but only when someone is psychotic and non-compos mentis can that be valid.

We need to remember that health is physical, mental, emotional, social and spiritual, whatever that might be to the person themselves. While we as health professionals are there to help, we become abusive when we try to take over the client's decisions that they have to live with for the rest of their life. We may not fully understand their decisions or even approve of them personally, but judgement is not ours to make. Our job is to support the client towards what they believe are the right choices for them.

At times, you may be faced with top-down and cross-wise decisions made by line managers, departmental policies and other care professionals, which you may be professionally or even contractually obliged to respect. This can put you in difficult and delicate positions if you think and believe those decisions are against the client's interests and well-being. It is important to remember how best we can facilitate the client's wants, needs and desires and use a decision tree to properly reflect these.

The Epidemic of Suicidal Thoughts

Over the years, many people who have transitioned and committed suicide were vastly underreported. They became long-term mentally dysfunctional patients who were simply unable to cope with the life that they were led to believe or convinced themselves was right for them. They were not taught the skills to survive as their destination identity. What ensued was long-term depression, personality disorders, schizoid breaks, long-term unemployment and addiction, with some ending up on a whole host of medications that dulled their ability to think. Many were parked in social housing and lived out their lives on state benefits. Even though many of those did not complete suicide, they could be plagued with constant thoughts of suicide.

Today we have an epidemic of people who started transition with the belief it would relieve them of their life problems. They often modelled themselves on the people who have publicly declared transition had rescued their life by living as their authentic self. They had not, however, reflected on how such a move would affect their own lives and end up not having the coping skills to live the life of the person they modelled. The reality of living the life as a person from a SGD group or transitioning from an already-established identity can be very much more complex and harder than initially perceived.

Unfortunately, we now also have therapists with very little or no experience in this field handing out referral letters like confetti in order to be perceived as doing the right thing or to make extra income from clients they do not know how to care for. The client is not doing the work they need to do psychologically and psychotherapeutically to manage their lives, goes into crisis, becomes depressed and suicidal, and sometimes retransitions back and forth multiple times having endless surgeries and procedures.

So many therapists do not understand the need for the clients to look at all their options by working with decision trees to probe the possible and probable outcomes of their thought patterns, decisions and outcomes. Neither do many therapists warn their clients of the pitfalls that come with those possible chosen directions in life and encourage preparation of strategies to be resilient.

Some people will find their way back from the North Pole blindfolded with their feet tied together. They are naturally and practised resilient people; no matter what you throw at them, they will get back up and carry on to success in whatever they do. This includes some people from SGD groups but certainly not all.

Not everyone has these resilient coping abilities. Perhaps they have been damaged by life or did not experience positive reinforcement during nurturing in childhood. They take life's blows much harder, and therapists treating these people need to train them to be more resilient and emotionally stronger when they hit the bumps and potholes on life's road. Therapy is not just talking to people from SGD groups about their feelings. Rather, it is helping them to manoeuvre their life and environment to help them avoid depression and suicidal thoughts.

Confabulation

One of the major problems that we as clinicians face when caring for people is the occurrence of confabulation. The idea that memory or experience is static and constant is not realistic. We know from research that stress affects the way we code memory traces. When memory is re-encoded, it can change (Deffenbacher et al., 2004). So, for most of us when we re-remember something 40 times, we remember 40 variations of those facts.

Some people have Highly Superior Autobiographical Memory (HSAM), a form of memory that is extraordinarily accurate, but these people are rare and not the average person (Park et al., 2016). For most of us, when we are re-encoding memory, that re-encoding takes place in many different parts of the brain and differently each time we recode. It is one of our survival mechanisms that helps us adapt to an ever-changing world.

When those memories, such as unwanted medical treatments or the frustration of lack of treatments, re-emerge with strong emotional feelings attached, stress occurs. This can retraumatise those clients when they recall the memories, and that in itself can distort the accuracy of the memory, affecting the adaptive survival mechanisms.

Also, as human beings, we change our memories in real-time to suit and adapt to a situation in the moment; that is, we confabulate (Brown et al., 2018). It is a survival strategy, but when people present to clinicians and health professionals, we are unclear at times that we are hearing accurate information from the client. As clinicians, we have to try to get the most accurate information we can for us to find the right ways to help people.

The more someone repeats what they tell other people, the more they believe it themselves, so people can end up convincing themselves something is true that never happened. They can convince themselves they belong to SGD groups by simply repeating that continual re-encoded information. When clinicians are not continually testing clients for the accuracy and congruency of that information, clinical mistakes can be made by issuing referral letters and recommending treatment and surgery that may not be right for that person, and ultimately, the patient has to pay the price.

There is also the issue that patients can purposefully lie and make things up when presenting to clinics. They learn "the script" of what to say to clinicians to get hormones and surgery. What they are presenting to clinics is a fabrication of someone else's story, who came before them, who used that story to get what they thought was the treatment they wanted.

The patient will often edit their own histories, make things up, outright lie and steal histories from other people to get the treatments they want. They can lie about medications they are taking, whether they have drug or alcohol issues, diseases, medical conditions or have had previous surgery. Sometimes a clinician will go along with this in order to get the fee and get the patient out of the door so they can move onto the next customer.

However, this is dangerous because clinics are being asked to make clinical decisions based on fiction. This does not allow the clinical process to deal with that person's situation and help them find really useful solutions that are specific to that person. The ramifications later are that the wrong clinical decision can be made, and the patient is left with the consequences of poor medical and surgical outcomes, even, at times, death from surgery, hormone administration or suicide.

Outside Influences

One of the major causes that contribute to clinical mistakes is the result of outside influences and pressures from other clinicians, healthcare workers, relatives and friends of the client from a SGD group. When it comes to the trajectory of a patient's health and direction in of their life, everyone can have an opinion. Some of those opinions may be well-informed, while others may be speculation or emotional blackmail.

Sometimes clinicians with different opinions and belief systems try to interfere with treatments. GPs of certain religious persuasions may try to get families to pressure the patient to withdraw from clinical care. They go far beyond their remit to manipulate the patient into stopping hormone treatment or having surgery, professing they know more about the patient than the specialist and convince families to withhold support. They may even lie to the family about the effectiveness and dangers of treatment or the legitimacy of the clinician.

Under this pressure and scare tactics, a patient may withdraw from the treatment programs, sinking into a deep depression but not wishing to lose their family. This is particularly prevalent in young people who have not yet fully formed their ability to make independent decisions apart from their family of origin.

They often feel isolated and railroaded but unable to exert their own will. In some cases, they are forced into seeing religious-based therapists and counsellors to correct their supposed "sinful" ways or even undergo conversion therapy. The depression experienced can lead to constant suicidal obsession. That depression may last for years until they finally break free from the influences of the family or at times attempt or complete suicide.

Sometimes partners or spouses seek to stop treatment. They may write angry, insulting letters to the clinicians, clinics, hospitals, or appeal to other clinicians for support and bring official complaints against the treating clinician in order to try to gain control of the situation. They may not want any part of family therapy or to learn how to accommodate the patient's treatment. The only agenda they are operating on or can see is their own.

This can also happen with parents of patients who do not want their offspring to seek any kind of help or only the kind of help that serves the parents' agenda. They will tell the clinician they do not believe that anyone is other than male or female and sex and gender diversity is a lot of old nonsense made up by unbalanced people and quacks. They have strong opinions and are dominators who rarely listen to their offspring, even if the patient's life is at risk.

Sometimes the client will break free and cut contact with those parents and sometimes they are not strong enough to do so and will continue to suffer the repeated abuse of the parent because it is all they know. They may comply with the parent's demands and have a deep underlying sense of low self-worth and are at high risk of suicide. The clinician can point out the dangers to the patient but are unable to interfere unless the patient speaks out and says they want help and want social services, other family members or the community to become involved.

It is a difficult situation because sometimes withdrawing a child from the home may cause more problems than the child waiting until they are of age and maturity to make their own decisions, but leaving them in such a situation runs the risk of suicide. There are even parents who would rather see their offspring dead than to deal with their sex and gender issues.

Decision Trees

Regardless of your discipline, you are likely to be familiar with decision trees, a tool you can use to make those difficult decisions so you can avoid, as much as possible, clinical mistakes and even get clients involved in decision-making processes (Goetz, 2011). Writing these out and weighing up the possible and probable outcomes helps you externalise and clarify your internal cognitions, observation, planned course of action and treatment plan.

Reflectively working with other professionals in case conferences or supervision can add layers of clarification that are unlikely to be achieved alone (Ozcan, 2017). Of course, time, case loads and funding are always our enemies, but in difficult cases where suicide risk is high, it is wise to take the extra time to use a decision tree.

Be sure to keep a record in your notes, dated, of the process, so should a clinical mistake occur or you are accused of negligence, you can show the trail of careful decision-making and professionalism. When using decision trees, be careful to use multiple recorded sources of information about the client so you can reach a balanced decision on how to proceed with that client.

We are living in a world of high accountability, lawsuits (particularly if you practise in America or Canada) and complaints. Since we will deal with many clients who have mental health problems, it is likely we will all have complaints made against us at some stage, justified or not. Some of us may also encounter opportunistic nuisance lawsuits from time to time when lawyers convince clients to sue, knowing that insurance companies would rather pay out a settlement than go to court. Those lawyers make a living out of a percentage of settlement fees. For all these reasons, keep fastidious notes.

Deadnaming

Deadnaming is the act of referring to someone who has changed their identity or claimed what they believe is their real identity, by a previous name. Under some anti-discrimination laws, it is illegal. Health carers deadnaming their client can damage the carer-client relationship, be psychologically wounding, breach privacy, destroy rapport and may actually be clinical negligence.

It may happen accidentally when someone is careless, on purpose when the person using the name refuses to recognise the person's change or officially when professionals are not being diligent in the way they are referring to their clients. Journalists use dead names when they are seeking to write sensational stories for clickbait, and trolls on the internet also use deadnaming to insult or harm people from a SGD group.

Some family members, particularly if they have extreme religious or philosophical views, do not accept a client's right to assert their own sense of self. They purposefully, continually and abusively refer to the client as their former name or natal registered sex or gender that the client has abandoned. When in conference with these relatives or other professionals, a health professional must respectfully refer to the client as they wish to be referred to, whether the family member or other professional accepts that identity or not. It may be awkward but the health professional must persist to respect the client's wishes first.

Legally, in recordkeeping and for accessing health fund benefits, where clients' documents may be in a different name, you may have to use the A.K.A (also known as) process in order to access notes or funds. You should, however, only do this with the client's permission and as soon as possible change the client's relevant documents and the file name, again with the client's permission.

The evolving field of clinical practice means that we experience many changes in processes, procedures and protocols during our careers in helping SGD groups. That evolution is driven by the availability of treatment, funding, shifting professional boundaries, departmental policy, research, the law and societal trends.

During the course of our practice, we fine-tune and hone our skills, so we all change the ways we practise as our careers advance. There is a fine line between negligence and a clinical accident, therefore we need to be mindful of that division. The first denotes culpability and the second is circumstances beyond clinical control.

Intersex campaigners have put forward proposed guidelines, such as the Australian and Aotearoa/New Zealand Intersex Organisation's Darlington Statement (2017). Unfortunately, these can tend to be exclusive and refer to people who are notedly born intersex, not accepting that people can be sex diverse in many ways or become intersex later in life.

The World Professional Association of Transgender Health (WPATH) publishes updated Standards of Care (2012).

This is an American text that frequently does not translate to other cultures and is generally out-of-date when it is published. Many countries now have their own versions, but again, they are limited in their application to real-life clinical practice where decisions must occasionally deviate from those guidelines to meet clients' specific needs.

To avoid negligence in suicide prevention with SGD people, it is prudent to constantly update your clinical skills and be aware of the political and social circumstances that affect the client's worldview.

Cultural Appropriation

As professionals we see, perceive, assess, manipulate and treat within our practices according to our training, informed doctrine, social gestalts, disciplinary codes of ethics and legal frameworks. These are, however, only our worldview and not necessarily reality, which is multi-dimensional according to who, what and where you are.

In each culture, there are people of sex and gender diversity whose reality is bound by their cultural world. So, it can be difficult for us to enter into other cultures and subgroups to deliver care. Those groups may not welcome outsiders or their input, health professionals included.

Abbey Stein (2020), who identifies as a transgender woman, was brought up as a first-born son in a closed Hasidic Jewish upstate New York Community. She is a direct descendant of Hasidic Judaism's founder, The Baal Shem Tov. Her father is a Rabbi and she did not learn English until she left the religion at 20 years of age.

Never having been on the internet, read newspapers or had anything other than a religious education, Stein knew nothing of transition until she left her community. Her father and ten siblings do not speak to her and she is excommunicated. A healthcare professional seeking to deliver suicide prevention care to a trans woman would not gain access to this community. Non-Orthodox professionals trying to enter this community to support SGD groups, telling the community to alter their beliefs, would be seen as, abusive, racist and offensive.

There are no figures for suicide of SGD people in Aboriginal and Torres Strait Islander communities but anecdotal community reports suggest suicides in the general Indigenous communities are more than twice the national average (Davidson, 2016). The problems of non-Aboriginal professionals trying to go onto country or into communities to deliver suicide prevention strategies is that they encounter complex issues around colonisation, which created layered oppression.

In Australia Aboriginal people are still being culturally devastated by Western corporations, the Australian Government that steals their lands and mining companies that poison their rivers. They face extreme racism, intergenerational trauma and a push for cultural assimilation. Not only is it difficult to deliver health services to these groups but also the health services that non-Aboriginal people try to deliver may not be culturally appropriate. Being a Brotherboy or Sistergirl in these cultures has a spiritual aspect that Western science fails to understand or knows how to address.

In delivering services cross-culturally in all countries, we run into many filters and barriers that we as clinicians may not be able to cross. If we push beyond cultural acceptability, we offend. It is always a better idea to try and offer assistance via open, diplomatic routes into these cultures, such as setting up culturally-appropriate suicide prevention through internal participation in the culture. Some people reach outside their cultures to gain clinical assistance. Always remember that the suicide recovery client may need at some time to reintegrate in harmony back into their culture once again.

We must always be aware of our privilege when working with clients and never assume that the client may have our advantages, whether they be physical, mental, emotional, social, educational or economic.

So, our decision-making brings us back to common sense, caution, kindness, valuing the client's needs for self-determination, pursuing the best interests of the client and protecting ourselves as practitioners. That does not always fit into rules, regulations, guidelines or doctrine, but it has to involve enthusiastically promoting the will to live in the way that is right for the client.

References

American Psychiatric Association. (1980). *DSM-III: Diagnostic and statistical manual of mental disorders.* Author.

Australian and Aotearoa/New Zealand Intersex Organisations. (2017). *Darlington Statement.* Retrieved from https://ihra.org.au/darlington-statement/

Brown, J., Huntley, D. & Morgan, S. (2018). Confabulation: etiology, typology, and intervention. *Clinical Research in Neurology.* 1(1). Retrieved from https://asclepiusopen.com/clinical-research-in-neurology/volume-1-issue-1/7.pdf

Cockerham, W. (2013). *Medical sociology on the move: New directions in theory.* Springer.

Davidson, H. (2016, May 5). No data exists on suicide among gay and trans indigenous Australian. *The Guardian.* Retrieved from https://www.theguardian.com/australia-news/2016/may/05/no-data-exists-on-suicide-among-gay-and-trans-indigenous-australians

Deffenbacher, K., Bornstein, B., Penrod, S. & McGorty, E. (2004). A meta-analytic review of the effects of high stress on eyewitness memory. *Law and Human Behavior, 28*(6), 687–706. Retrieved from https://link.springer.com/article/10.1007/s10979-004-0565-x

Goetz, T. (2011). *The decision tree: How to make better choices and take control of your health* (1st ed). Rodale Books.

Hinkle, S. (2019, January 27). Utah lawmakers want to make it impossible to correct gender markers. *Instinct Magazine.* Retrieved from https://instinctmagazine.com/utah-lawmakers-want-to-make-it-impossible-to-correct-gender-markers/

Laing, R.D., & Esterson, A. (1964). *Sanity, madness and the family.* Penguin Books.

Murphy, P. (2019, June 21). A psychoanalysts group long said gay and trans people were abnormal. Now it's apologizing for those views. *CNN.* Retrieved from https://edition.cnn.com/2019/06/21/health/gay-trans-apology-disorder-trnd/index.html

New International Version. (2011). *Bible Hub.* Retrieved from: https://biblehub.com/niv/matthew/19.htm

Ozcan, Y. (2017). *Analytics and decision support in health care operations management* (3rd ed). Jossey-Bass Public Health.

Park, E., Cahill, L. & McGaugh J. (2006). A case of unusual autobiographical remembering. *Neurocase*, 12(1), 35–49. Retrieved from https://www.ncbi.nlm.nih.gov/pubmed/16517514

Stein, A. (2020). *Becoming Eve: My journey from ultra-orthodox rabbi to transgender woman.* Seal Press.

Szasz, T. (2007). *Coercion as cure: A critical history of psychiatry.* Transaction Publishers.

Washington, A. (2017, August 17). Arnold Schwarzenegger slams Trump: "There are not two sides to hatred." *The Hollywood Reporter.* Retrieved from https://www.hollywoodreporter.com/news/arnold-schwarzenegger-tells-trump-are-not-two-sides-hatred-1030788

World Health Organization (WHO). (1998). *International Statistical Classification of Diseases and Related Health Problems (ICD)*. Retrieved from https://www.who.int/classifications/icd/ICD10Volume2_en_2010.pdf

Chapter 7:
Reasons for Suicide

Knight (2017) reports that many paediatricians have repeatedly been advising parents of intersex children born with non-stereotypical genitals to allow the child to be operated on to cosmetically normalise their genitals. This is driven by the myth that making them appear stereotypically male or female will avoid the child being a misfit and completing suicide later in life. These statements, as mentioned previously however, have no grounds in science or evidence to back them up.

It is clear in many cases that the opposite is true in that some intersex people may regret the surgery ever having been done as they try to negotiate what they believe is their true sex or identity of being intersex in its own right. Intersex civil rights organisations advise it is better to allow the child to decide how their body needs to be as they grow up and negotiate their own identity.

By forcing the child to conform to the so-called norm, it is teaching them shame around their body and so can give them a sense of sex dysphoria, a feeling of not being valid or right in their body. When we consider that there is at least the same number of red-haired people in the world as there are officially recognised intersex people, plus many more sex-variant people, we must ask ourselves, would we dye the hair of a red-haired child so they fit into society?

There are indeed intersex children who need emergency surgery when born to allow their bodies to metabolically function well, but for the majority, there is no functional reason to operate on them at such an early age, without their prior permission. Parents, however, are scared and panicked into allowing surgery when paediatricians strongly push them towards that decision.

The BBC (McDermott, 2018) reported an interview with 23-year-old Anick who was born intersex, in India, with genitals that did not resemble either male or female. Anick said he had seen over 100 clinicians in the last few years in a quest to get a surgeon to build him a penis. As a child, he was taken to see doctors every six months who would use words like "abnormal" and "atypical". While he felt loved by his parents, Anick knew he was different even though people told him he was just like other boys. He found it hard to make friends at school and would hold his breath in an attempt to suffocate himself. After a more serious suicide attempt at 14 years of age, he was given counselling.

Anick said, "I didn't want anyone else to know who didn't need to know. It was very, very isolating." He thought no one knew what was different about him and that he was the only person like himself in the world. Discovering there were other people like him made a huge difference in that he thought he did not have to be ashamed of who he was and the way he was born. Doctors told him he could start considering penile construction at 18 so he decided to tell other people to prepare them for the many operations he would be undergoing. The Organisation Intersex International (OII) 2018 Conference in Copenhagen was the first time he had ever met other intersex people and the first time he felt he did not need to explain himself to other people.

In the documentary *Secret Intersex: Neither Boy Nor Girl* (Channel 4, 2017), Steph, who lives as a male but was born with Klinefelter's Syndrome, talked about how a lack of genital development as a male, small testes and a micropenis nearly drove him to suicide. For him, puberty arrived at 27 when he was finally diagnosed and started testosterone therapy. While he lives as a male, he says he feels like both sexes.

An anonymous intersex suicide survivor posted the following on an intersex activist site (Marquez, 2010):

"I may seem like a strong person, but in reality, I am fragile deep inside; you have no clue to my daily battles, you have no clue what it's like to be in my skin. When people treat me different I feel it deep within and though I shouldn't let things get to me, they do, for I have to fight every day to be just me. When people see only my disability and disorders, you fail to see that I am just as good a human being like anyone else."

Hong Kong Intersex campaigner Small Luk, born with Partial Androgyne Insensitivity Syndrome (PAIS), talks about how she was brought up as a boy and underwent over 20 surgeries (Chan, 2020). Unsuccessful surgeries, bullying and constant pressure from her family to live as the first-born male drove her to attempt suicide twice.

When she was born, doctors classified her as male. Confused about why she was to undergo so many surgeries, she eventually rejected submitting herself to those operations. Developing breasts as a teenager, she started to bleed each month. It was only at 36 that an examination revealed underdeveloped female reproductive organs. Although she holds a female ID card, she considers herself intersex and says society needs to accept intersex differences as variations in nature, not diseases.

Katharine Prescott appeared on CNN (2017) talking about her 14-year-old trans child Kyler who took their own life after having transitioned from girl to boy at school. It seemed he had been bullied online, which brought on deep depression that led to his suicide.

He dressed and presented as a boy but was caught up in the US political row where the right-wing wanted trans children to use the bathroom of their birth registration. He was the third trans teen to complete suicide within a few months in the San Diego area.

At this time many American children from SGD groups feel highly insecure and unsafe going to school. The bathroom row has made them into misfits within an education system that does not respect their right to exist. This leads to high levels of anxiety and depression with an increase in suicidal thoughts, and attempted and successful suicides.

Florida woman Patricia McKay Verbeeck, mother of a trans teenager, shared the suicide story of her child, Eric Peter Verbeeck (Hahn, 2018), who suicided when about to graduate. Eric was registered male at birth but had already begun transition to female. Eric had commenced oestrogen hormone therapy and was waiting to move after graduation in order to present as female in public.

Eric jumped from the 12th floor of their building to their death. They wrote about the pain and hopelessness they felt, even having been accepted into several colleges. Their sense of utter hopelessness about their future is common among many teenagers from SGD groups, who are just struggling to be schoolkids.

Eric wrote:

"I would like to be remembered as a transgendered, pansexual, teenage girl named Hope. Being transgender is my identity. My sexual orientation or identity is being pansexual, meaning I do not care about what the person is; I care about who they are. Sexual orientation is about who you go to bed with and gender is about who you go to bed as."

Justine Newell (CTV News, 2017), a 13-year-old trans boy from Cape Breton, Canada, registered female at birth, took his life after experiencing an intense tirade of bullying. As an out trans teenage boy, the bullies would tell him to go kill himself and shoot himself in the face.

He had been out for a while and gave talks in schools about how it was okay to be different. He had spoken to his father about a friend who was suffering bullying and how he gave them tips to get past the assaults, but it seemed that the bullying he faced himself finally became too much for him.

It was the third child suicide in the area over a short period. It is important to note that when bullying in the community or online becomes prevalent, the bully tends to focus on people they believe are vulnerable. No matter how mature and intelligent a child from a SGD group may be, it is wise for carers and teachers to always remember they are vulnerable due to the nature of their very difference.

Seventeen-year-old Leelah Alcorn (Molloy, 2020), a trans female registered male at birth, announced to her parents that she believed she was transgender. Reportedly, they responded by telling her that she would never truly be a girl, that God does not make mistakes, and did not accept her. A few years later, she killed herself by stepping in front of a truck on an early Sunday morning three days after Christmas, after what she claimed was years of emotional abuse by her devout Christian parents.

In a post online, Leelah wrote that her parents had told her it was only a phase or fantasy. She explained that what was constantly said to her made her hate herself and believe that the life she had ahead was not worth living. In her suicide note, she said that her parents only took her to Christian therapists, repeatedly refusing to allow her to transition as a minor.

She wrote:

"My death needs to mean something. My death needs to be counted in the number of transgender people who commit suicide this year. I want someone to look at that number and say, 'That's fucked up' and fix it. Fix society, Please."

Evie MacDonald (Caines, 2019), an Australian child living as a boy, told her parents at nine years old that she would rather die than live as a boy. In an interview she said:

"I want to be a Princess and I want to play with Barbies [dolls], and watch all those movies and stuff. I knew that I was different. Inside I always felt like a girl but I just didn't know how to say that in words. I wrote 'I want to die' because for me it felt like I would rather go to heaven than live here as a boy. I snapped and I said, 'Why can't you just accept me as I am?' She [Evie's mother] came to me and said, 'Why do you want to die?' and I told her the reason and she goes 'Well, you know I'd rather have a daughter that is alive than a son that's dead'."

The mother Meagan MacDonald said in the interview:

"What I was doing by not supporting my child was actually worse. My kid was really struggling. If I didn't support Evie, I categorically know that Evie wouldn't be here. So she would have at least attempted suicide at least multiple times or even worse actually completed it."

A New South Wales coronial inquest in Australia into the death of Veronica Baxter, a 34-year-old Aboriginal trans woman, found she had completed suicide at Silverwater Men's Detention Facility in 2009 (Wood, 2011). Arrested a few days before at Sydney Gay and Lesbian Mardi Gras and charged with selling drugs, she had been placed in a men's facility and denied her prescribed hormone medication. Although she had lived for years as female, she had told a friend that if she found herself in that situation, she would not be able to cope and would end it all. Having been interviewed by two counsellors after her arrest, no one from correctional services identified her as being at risk of suicide nor took actions to isolate her or transfer her to a female facility.

Lucy Meadows, a trans woman who was transitioning on the job in a British primary school in 2013, suffered a barrage of public humiliation from the press (Smith, 2017). By all accounts, her colleagues reported she was an excellent teacher and well-liked by the children. She told the school she was transitioning and started back at the school as Miss Meadows. The school diplomatically sent letters out to all of the parents notifying them of the change, but a few parents objected; they started a harassment campaign and attracted interest from the national press.

Press and photographers harassed Meadows' family, offering them money for a story and began to write demeaning and humiliating articles about her. Meadows wrote to others about how, though she had done nothing wrong, she had to leave the house by the back door and arrive at school early to avoid the press. One particular reporter, Richard Littlejohn from *The Daily Mail*, wrote, "He's not only in the wrong body ... he's in the wrong job". Meadows experienced great emotional distress and she suicided.

At the inquest, the coroner for Blackburn, Hyndburn and Rossendale, Michael Singleton, singled out *The Daily Mail* for criticism. He commented that the paper had been guilty of "ridicule and humiliation" and "character assassination".

In 2015, Rachel Bryk, 23, completed suicide by jumping off the George Washington Bridge and into the Hudson river (Messing et al., 2015). Two nearby police tried to stop her and shouted for her not to do it, but she had reached her limit of tolerance. She left a message to appear on her Twitter after her death: "Guess I am dead. Killed myself. Sorry". Bryk's parents had no problems with her transition at age 22 and were glad she was happy.

Unfortunately, Bryk had experienced considerable bullying.

She wrote online, "The rest of you don't have to worry though, I'm going to kill myself soon enough and you won't have to be bothered by me anymore." A bully wrote back, "DO IT, if you're such a weak-willed, thin-skinned dips––t then f––king do it." Some people are not strong enough to stand up to bullies, particularly if they are from a SGD group, already suffering minority stress and having to deal with transition, which can be very stressful in and of itself.

A San Francisco-based transgender actress, comedienne and activist Daphne Dorman took her life in 2019. She posted on Facebook (Assunção, 2020):

> *"I've thought about this a lot before this morning. How do you say 'goodbye' and 'I'm sorry' and 'I love you' to all the beautiful souls you know? For the last time. To those of you who are mad at me: please forgive me. To those of you who wonder if you failed me: you didn't. To those of you who feel like I failed you: I did and I'm sorry and I hope you'll remember me in better times and better light. I love you all. I'm sorry. Please help my daughter, Naia, understand that none of this is her fault. Please remind her that I loved her with every fiber of my being."*

Dorman had recently been referenced in a Netflix special by another comedian who told jokes about trans people that were widely criticised as being transphobic.

Amber Corbin, the wife of a transgender man, spoke out about the suicide of her husband. Corbin explained that not everyone accepted his transition and the bullying was relentless. In an interview, in tears, she told *WPSD Local 6* (Wife Speaks Out About Bullying, Education, 2020), "It played a big part in why I no longer have my husband." Just because someone has transitioned to male does not mean they have hardened and cease to be affected by constant criticism about their sex and gender status.

A trans woman, Madona Kiparoidze, tried to set herself on fire in front of City Hall in Tbilisi, Georgia, USA (Bollinger, 2020). She was protesting the state's response to trans people's needs during the COVID-19 lockdown. Police officers managed to pull her coat off her and then arrested her when she said, "I am a transgender woman, and I'm setting myself on fire because the Georgian state doesn't care about me."

Another protester commented, "We can't even pay for our rent. What can we do?" The state had a policy of not recognising trans people unless they have had genital surgery, which for many is outside of their economic capacity.

During the COVID-19 lockdown, a 38-year-old HIV-positive transgender woman in the Malvina area of Malad, Maharashtra, India, hanged herself due to her loss of livelihood and the unavailability of medicine (Struggling to Survive in Lockdown, 2020). Having run out of money, she found it hard to make ends meet. The lack of availability of medication for her condition pushed her over the edge and she found it too hard to survive, believing she would not survive anyway.

Many people from SGD groups throughout the world live on the margins of society in poverty, find it difficult to survive and are unable to afford medical care, particularly in developing countries.

A 22-year-old trans woman in Russia, Dasha Stern, reportedly suicided in 2013 when she was fired from her job because her employers feared they were in violation of a nationwide ban on "propaganda of nontraditional sexual relationships", put in place by President Putin (Brydum, 2020). Stern had also recently been disowned by her parents and thrown out of her home. She had been approved for a mortgage and car loan but was unable to make the payments when she lost her job.

The nationwide ban was mainly driven by homophobia but affected all people who may seem other than heteronormative. Just the perception of someone being other than heteronormative is enough to warrant harassment, mistreatment and exclusion from Russian society in general. While Russia, like many other republics throughout the Russian Federation, interacts with the World Health Organization, it rejects many of its human rights and health recommendations.

What is also important to remember is that the attacks on SGD groups of people and individuals also affect those around them. A 20-year-old man, Maurice Willoughby, who had recently made a video defending his relationship with his transgender girlfriend, was found dead shortly afterwards by suicide. His girlfriend said he died of an overdose after she left him. It is believed he was bullied after he went public about the relationship (Orso, 2020).

Suicide over gender also occurs in children and people who are less stereotypically gendered than the social norm (15-Yr-Old Boy Commits Suicide, 2018). In a private school at Chintamani in Tiruchirappalli, India, a 15-year-old student completed suicide by hanging himself after being teased for the way he acted and talked. Four other students, who have been charged by the local police, bullied him for having feminine mannerisms. The parents cited the teachers' and school's indifference around the boy's complaints about being bullied as the cause.

Kirk Murphy hanged himself at 38 years of age (Roberts, 2011). Perplexed by his death, deeper investigation by his sister revealed that their parents had sent Murphy to a government-funded experimental behavioural alteration program at UCLA to eradicate his effeminate mannerisms. His family believed the program, designed to purge the "sissy" out of him, changed him to the extent that he was never the same again, leaving him stricken with the belief that he was broken and different from everyone else. Murphy's sister reported that he was unable to connect with many other students for fear of judgment and that he ate his lunch in the boys' bathroom for three years during his senior schooling.

166

Murphy was treated by Dr George Rekers, who became an outspoken anti-gay rights campaigner who stated that homosexuality was an illness. He used a token economy system where Murphy was rewarded for stereotypically male behaviour and ignored and punished, including beatings, for feminine behaviour. Although Murphy went on to become a high-profile gay rights campaigner, his family believe that the early treatment permanently damaged him. Many years later, Dr Rekers was photographed arriving at Miami Airport with a male sex worker who he later described as his personal assistant but denied he was gay (*CNN*, 2010).

It would be impossible to engage in the discussion around suicidal ideation in SGD groups of people without also engaging in the meta-discussion around the enforcement of sex and gender stereotypes by patriarchy and misogyny driven by the men and women who enforce the social constrictions imposed by men.

A young lesbian couple—Tandel and Rujukta Gawand—from Suman Nagar, Chunabhatti Mumbai, India, engaged in suicide after their love affair was discovered by a parent who sought to separate them; one woman succeeded and one was taken to hospital (Abraham, 2020). Women in India and much of the world are often considered a possession of the dominant masculine state and philosophies. According to this viewpoint, to deviate from that ultra-feminine, heteronormative, subservient stereotype, which is meant to serve the male establishment, is not considered feminine and is to be corrected at all costs.

Little is known about suicide in butch-gendered women as it is poorly researched and recorded. What we know is that butches can experience prejudice and oppression from many directions such as misogyny, the heteronormative women who support misogyny, and lesbians who see being butch as an oppression of the feminine. Being a butch woman was fought for in the lesbian community in safe spaces like the Gateways Club in London which operated between 1931 and 1985 (Gardiner, 2003).

Label words like "butch", "dyke" and "drag king" could be used as insults but were reimagined by the queer community as badges of honour. Fourth-wave feminists have, however, at times sought to ban words like "dyke", perceiving it as an insult but not understanding how hard its ownership was fought for by their predecessors who paved the way for their liberties. Butches are often mistaken for trans people and asked when they are going to transition when they are simply comfortable living as butch women.

There is a largely silent population of people who cross-dress during sex or at home who typically do not appear in statistics. They are generally men but can include women, who have been traditionally referred to as transvestites and cross-dressers and are, to the greatest extent, in heterosexual relationships but can be bisexual, gay or omnisexual (O'Keefe, 2007). They do not associate with or refer to themselves as trans or transgendered. What they do is highly secretive and often not known to the public; in fact, they fear public disclosure of their habits.

If they are not in a relationship, they can visit sex workers or become subservient to a dominatrix. Their drive for cross-dressing is generally a sexually-driven fetish, and they experience no sex or gender dysphoria or desire in any way to live as a member of the opposite sex. Where they can become suicidal is when their partners are unable to accept and accommodate the fetish; this threatens the relationship to the point that the individual suddenly becomes consumed with extreme separation anxiety which can lead to suicide.

A meta-analysis of research data indicated that the loss of a perceived sense of masculinity in men who lose their testicles to cancer or trauma and had to undergo an orchidectomy, led to an increased (20%) rise of suicide compared to the general population (Alanee & Russo, 2012). While the public would be generally unaware of their medical condition, the suicidal individual obviously experiences a sense of sex dysphoria in feeling less than male.

In an individual-centred approach study of women with breast cancer, it was found that that suicidal ideation was two to seven times more prevalent than in general epidemiological studies (Güth et al., 2011). The trauma of the loss of breast tissue, as with the loss of testicles, can cause a profound alteration to self-image; this can lead to a sense of loss of confidence and the creation of sex dysphoria. While this study did not compensate for those who may experience metastasis, its results were significant.

Male history has and still does dominate female history, and when it is written, this is often done misogynistically towards women and feminine people. This also includes the recording of history in the queer community as women have less academic and economic power. Feminine people have frequently been and are redacted from history, economics, politics, religion, statistics and morality. So a major part of examining suicidal drivers in SGD groups is pulling back the curtain of patriarchal-driven research, classifications, systemic medical systems and perspectives.

Reasons for Suicidal Ideation and Suggested Targeted Interventions

→ **An existential crisis about the person's physical sex and/ or gender diversity status.**
Support self-exploration and accommodation of a person's right to be unique, regardless of perceived or constructed social norms.

→ **Rejection by partners, family and friends.**
Education around systemic interpersonal relationships and how to negotiate the world as a mature independent individual on one's own terms.

→ Ostracisation and demonisation from religious and right-wing groups, including exclusion from educational establishments or work opportunities.
Fostering understanding that all religions and societies can have a profuse spectrum of belief systems, many of which freely accept people of sex or gender diversity. Educating the client that religious or social extremism is not necessarily about the client personally. Fostering a drive to persistently seek opportunities where they can.

→ Traumatic stress and post-traumatic stress due to non-consensual or coercive medical procedures and lack of available or approachable healthcare, including endocrinology, surgery, mental health services and social support.
Finding peer group support from other individuals in the same situation with whom the client shares experiences and can glean support through social media and face-to-face contact. Asking for solutions from professionals and peer support groups.

→ Homelessness, insecure accommodation issues and experiences of living in an area or culture where the person may experience constant potential threats, harassment and violence.
Introducing the client to the social services including public housing departments. Encouraging the client to be proactive in taking their personal safety into their own hands by being part of community-based citizens' safety programs, in coordination with the local police if possible or safe to do so.

→ Difficulty in finding work, being deselected from career ladders and being unjustly fired due to sex and/or gender diversity prejudice.
Connecting the client to employment, legal and political services that may assist them in finding a remedy without

overly enthusing about justice.

→ **A sense of isolation, loneliness, depression and imposed economic disadvantage in accordance with minority stress theory.**
Teach life and social skills, treating the depression and introducing the client to archetypes of people who transcended minority isolation, including examples of people from SGD groups.

→ **Regrets from having transitioned their physical body to represent another sex or regrets from having lived as a different gender other than they were raised as a child.**
This tends to come about when people have been pushed into a diagnosis of sex and/or gender dysphoria by clinicians, following unrealistic expectations of what transition can offer, or have undergone medical procedures as an infant without their consent. The client needs to be helped to explore living as the person they feel is the most comfortable for them.

→ **Bullying, rejection and ostracisation within SGD groups. Since such groups can contain emotionally wounded people, vilification can occur when people do not fit in. There can be considerable bullying around forcing people to describe themselves by certain labels that are not comfortable for them. This seems particularly prevent online and on social media platforms.**
Teaching the person to live the majority of their lives in society and not just retreating to sub-culture support groups that they may have come to depend on for approval of their lived experience.

→ **Mental health issues that might be outside the professional competence of a treating clinician.**
Cross-referral to appropriate health professionals.

Of course, there are other reasons someone from a SGD group may complete or consider suicide that I have not mentioned here. They may include suicidal drivers that have nothing to do with the person's sex and/or gender diversity. As health professionals, we seek out those reasons when we can so we can help devise a rescue plan. Some clients, however, can confabulate for many reasons when they do not want to disclose or admit their reasons for contemplating suicide.

We must tread a fine line between observation, questioning, probing, analysis and becoming intrusive. We can constantly and carefully tread this line by always putting the needs of the client first above any other interested parties including relatives, partners or other professionals, while still fulfilling our own professional duties.

As well as showing many of the reasons here for suicidal ideation in SGD groups and people experiencing sex and/or gender dysphoria and variance, we must also consider unseen or hidden influences. With many clients, we may never know the real drivers that push them to consider or attempt suicide.

As professionals and human beings, we should always keep in mind that we are also part of the problem. We come to the client with our own preconceived ideas and perceptions of what sex and gender might or might not be, which at the end of the day, are just our own constructs and not necessarily concrete facts.

References

15-yr-old boy commits suicide after friends tease his behaviour as feminine. (2018, February 9). *Deccan Chronicle*. Retrieved from https://www.deccanchronicle.com/nation/current-affairs/090218/15-yr-old-tamil-nadu-boy-suicide-classmates-tease-behaviour-feminine-c

Abraham, B. (2016, August 31). Mumbai lesbian couple attempts suicide after family spot them together in beach, one dies. *India Times*. Retrieved from https://www.indiatimes.com/news/india/ mumbai-lesbian-couple-attempts-suicide-after-family-spot-them-together-one-dies-260907.html

Alanee S. & Russo, P. (2012). Suicide in men with testis cancer. *European Journal of Cancer Care (England)*. Retrieved from https://www.ncbi.nlm.nih.gov/ pubmed/22624649

Assunção, M. (2019, October 12). Transgender actress, activist and comedienne Daphne Dorman, referenced in Dave Chappelle's 'transphobic' Netflix special, commits suicide. *New York Daily News*. Retrieved from https://www. nydailynews.com/news/national/ny-daphne-dorman-dave-chappelle-suicide-transphobic-netflix-special-20191012-kbwfswhydjgalp4mro2hcmvpxm-story.html

Bollinger, A. (2020, May 1). Trans woman sets herself on fire to protest government's poor COVID-19 response. *LGBTQ Nation*. Retrieved from https://www.lgbtqnation. com/2020/05/trans-woman-sets-fire-protest-govern-ments-poor-covid-19-response/

Brydum, S. (2013, October 22). Trans woman commits suicide after firing under Russia's 'propaganda' ban. *The Advocate*. Retrieved from https://www.advocate.com/politics/ transgender/2013/10/22/trans-woman-commits-suicide-after-firing-under-russias-propaganda

Caines, Kimberley. (2019, January 9). 'I'd rather go to heaven than live here as a boy': Inside the lives of Australian trans children. *9 News*. Retrieved from https:// www.9news.com.au/2019/01/29/10/23/transgender-news-australia-child-self-harm-and-mental-health

Chan, H. (2017, May 8). The Hong Kong intersex campaigner who's tearing down barriers. *South China Morning*

Post. Retrieved from https://www.scmp.com/news/ hong-kong/education-community/article/2093440/ hong-kong-intersex-campaigner-whos-tearing-down

Channel 4, Real Stories. (2017). *Secret intersex: born genderless* [Medical Documentary]. Retrieved from https:// www.youtube.com/watch?v=reilipcN4_Y&has_verified=1

CNN. (2017, February 23). Mom of transgender teen who took his life speaks out. Retrieved from https://www.youtube. com/watch?v=EA0nb_lCG-g

CNN Wire Staff. (2010, May 14). Anti-gay rights activist resigns after trip with male escort. Retrieved from http://edition.cnn.com/2010/US/05/12/anit.gay.activist. resigns/index.html

CTV News. (2017, June 24). Cape Breton family speaking out about trans-teen's suicide. Retrieved from https://www. youtube.com/watch?v=11fqoY7eQk0

Gardiner, J. (2003). *From the closet to the screen: Women at the Gateways Club 1945–85.* Pandora Books.

Güth, U., Myrick M.E., Reisch T., Bosshard, G. & Schmid, S.M. (2011). Suicide in breast cancer patients: An individual-centered approach provides insight beyond epidemiology. *Acta Oncologica*, 50(7), 1037-1044. Retrieved from https://www.ncbi.nlm.nih.gov/ pubmed/21861596

Hahn, J.D. (2018, March 16). Mom shares transgender teen's heartbreaking suicide note to raise awareness to issues she faced. *People.* Retrieved from https://people.com/ human-interest/transgender-teen-suicide-note/

Knight, K. (2017, September 10). If a doctor tells a parent that surgery could prevent their child's suicide, it's not true. *Huffington Post.* Retrieved from https://www.hrw.org/

news/2017/09/10/if-doctor-tells-parent-surgery-could-prevent-their-childs-suicide-its-not-true

Marquez, A.R. (2017, August 3). An anonymous message from a suicidal intersex survivor [Blog post]. Retrieved from https://anunnakiray.com/2017/08/03/an-anonymous-message-from-a-suicidal-intersex-survivor/

McDermott, S. (2018, October 26). My intersex life: Now I have a new penis, I hope I will find love. *BBC Stories.* Retrieved from www.bbc.com/news/stories-45979431

Messing, P., Sauchelli, D. & Fears, D. (2015, April 29). Bullying behind transgender woman's leap off bridge. *New York Post.* Retrieved from https://nypost.com/2015/04/29/bullying-behind-transgender-womans-leap-off-bridge/

Molloy, A. (2015, January 1). Leelah Alcorn: Transgender teenager's parents 'should be prosecuted', says gay rights activist. *The Independent.* Retrieved from https://www.independent.co.uk/news/world/americas/leelah-alcorn-transgender-teenagers-parents-should-be-prosecuted-says-gay-rights-activist-9952742.html

O'Keefe, T. (2007). *Autogynephilia and autoandrophilia in non-sex and gender dysphoric persons.* Paper presented at the World Association for Sexual Health conference, Sydney, Australia. Retrieved from https://tracieokeefe.com/autogynephilia-and-autoandrophilia-in-non-sex-and-gender-dysphoric-persons/

Orso, A. (2019, August 22). Philadelphia man dies by suicide after video goes viral of him defending relationship with trans girlfriend, friends say. *The Philadelphia Inquirer.* Retrieved from https://www.inquirer.com/news/maurice-willoughby-died-by-suicide-after-viral-video-defending-transgender-girlfriend-20190822.html

Roberts, F. (2011, June 10). Family blame UCLA 'sissy boy' therapy by anti-gay professor for death of their effeminate son. *The Daily Mail, Australia.* Retrieved from https://www.dailymail.co.uk/news/article-2000529/Family-lame-UCLA-sissy-boy-therapy-anti-gay-professor-sons-suicide.html

Smith, R. (2017, November 19). Lucy Meadows was a transgender teacher who took her own life. Her story must be remembered. *The Independent.* Retrieved from https://www.independent.co.uk/news/long_reads/lucy-meadows-transgender-teacher-ruth-smith-media-press-daily-mail-lgbt-rights-a8063946.html

Struggling to survive in lockdown transgender kills self. (2020, May 12). *National Herald.* Retrieved from https://www.nationalheraldindia.com/national/struggling-to-survive-in-lockdown-transgender-kills-self

Wife speaks out about bullying, education after transgender husband commits suicide. (2019, November 3). *WPSD Local 6.* Retrieved from https://www.wpsdlocal6.com/wife-speaks-out-about-bullying-education-after-transgender-husband-commits/video_ce06cdfe-febf-11e9-b424-73c07dd41289.html

Wood, A. (2011, April 10). 'Why did our sister die in a men's jail?' *Sydney Morning Herald.* Retrieved from https://www.smh.com.au/national/nsw/why-did-our-sister-die-in-a-mens-jail-20110409-1d8fe.html

Chapter 8:
Establishing Norms for Sex and/or Gender Diverse Groups of People

One of the most fascinating developments in the field of sex and gender diversity is the speed at which it has changed over the past 25 years since the widespread introduction of the internet. The clinical, legal and social language we used then now seems archaic.

At that time, the intersex movement had little exposure publicly except for some academic publications in medicine and sociology and a few autobiographies like those of Georgina Somerset (Turtle, 1963), Dawn Langley-Simmons (1995) and Lady Colin Campbell (1997). Any intersex person who spoke out was considered to be breaking ranks because clinicians had expressly told them not to talk about their issues to others. They had to keep their secret.

Erik Schinegger, who was registered female at birth in Austria and raised as a female named Erika, was the world champion women's downhill skier in 1966 (Man Who Won '66 Women's Downhill Gives up Medal, 2015). During a genetic screening, it was discovered Erika had a Y chromosome and further investigation found a full set of male reproductive organs that had grown inside instead of developing outside the body. Doctors for the skiing association tried to convince Erika to undergo surgery to remove all those organs to avoid a public scandal and the impression that she had cheated in winning the women's medal. They tried to keep the truth about the extent of Erik's male sex organs from him.

Erika had always appeared quite masculine for a girl and

enjoyed many stereotypically outdoor boys' pursuits although she grew up believing she was female but never developed breasts or menstruated. Fortunately, a nun and urologist persuaded her that the surgery to remove her male organs would be wrong. The urologist performed surgery to free the male sex organs. Erik changed to living as a man at 19 years old, went on to marry twice, fathered a daughter, ran one of Austria's biggest ski schools and gave the women's medal back years later.

British woman Suzy Temko talked about how she was diagnosed with complete AIS at age 16 and told by the doctor not to tell anyone (Gizauskas, 2019). Suzy had fallen over at a party a few weeks earlier and found a lump in her midriff. She was operated on for stage four cancer and during the surgery, the surgeons discovered her ovaries were actually testicles, which were removed.

Reflecting at 27, she said, "I wanted to tell people. It was a misguided idea by the doctors to protect me, and I understand where they were coming from as society sees people who are different as unfavourable. But all that did was reinforce that being intersex was wrong or bad. The shame and the stigma reinforced that I needed to hide."

When Temko got malaria, a doctor insisted she was a boy and should describe herself as having a boy's body even though she had lived her life as female, was registered as female at birth and looked like an ordinary female with a vagina. She was so upset by the way she had been treated that she began experiencing an eating order and suicidal thoughts.

In many parts of the world, intersex people are still treated as imposters by legal systems and doctors who fail to listen to them. Many medics believe that they have the right to determine what sex a person can present as and what medical procedures they should undergo. Many intersex people are happy with the decisions doctors made for them, but more are coming forward who campaign for the right for intersex people to define themselves as male, female, intersex or whatever they feel is right for them. They want to be recognised physically and legally as they see fit.

The introduction of the diagnosis of Disorders of Sexual Development (DSD) to replace the word 'intersex' has caused great dissatisfaction among many intersex people (Interact, 2016). It denotes wrongness and many intersex people find it unnecessarily stigmatising when they might not need or want medical intervention. They believe it seeks to erase recognition of being intersex.

The Council of Europe Commissioner for Human Rights published an issues paper on the experiences of intersex people and how they are treated (Council of Europe, 2015). On 14 February 2019 The European Parliament adopted its first resolution dedicated to intersex human rights. It further brought to light the prejudices and violence perpetrated against intersex people and set out initial pathways for European states to change laws to protect this population (The EU Parliament's LGBTI Intergroup, 2019). The resolution took a clear position against the medicalisation and pathologisation of intersex people, and was opposed to sex-normalising treatments and surgeries, without prior informed consent of the person themselves.

Previously, trans issues were very much controlled in Western culture by the dogma of the Harry Benjamin International Gender Dysphoria Association (Meyer et al., 2002) and were wholly concerned with the processes of transsexuals transitioning from male to female or vice versa. The Standards of Care were guidelines by which clinicians should practise and recommended for best clinical outcomes. Those of us as practitioners who strayed from those standards to suit the client's needs could come under attack from the establishment, particularly psychiatry, which comprised predominantly white, privileged, patriarchal males, often with academic tenure as well as senior hospital positions.

The fringe was the cross-dresser community who were still considered to be suffering from a fetish, paraphilia, and could be tolerated as long as they were not involved too much with public exhibitionism. To turn up dressed as another sex or gender to a corporate event would have run the risk of being turned away, cited as behaving unsuitably and sometimes getting fired.

There were very few people who were talking about being androgynous or having a sense of identifying as no sex or gender. They were considered academic curiosities. Many clinicians were just puzzled by anyone who did not want to be seen as either male or female or even anyone who did not want to be heteronormative.

Most academics or clinicians knew nothing or virtually nothing about intersex or gender variations like bissu, Hijra, khushra, Kathoey, fa'afafine, bakla, muxe, Native American gender structures, Albanian sworn virgins living as male, third inuit girl child raised as male, the New York Ball culture, drag queens, butches, or those who lived sometimes as male and sometimes as female.

From an academic and medical perspective, from the early part of the 20th century until the birth of the internet, the norm officially was heteronormative. Anyone who did not fit that paradigm was to be fixed either by therapy or as a last resort by hormonal alteration and surgery so they would fit into the heteronormative model.

Two things changed everything. The first was the free flow of information via the internet. Knowledge that had previously been the exclusive domain of the medical profession and locked away in libraries, which the public could often not access, was suddenly available at the stroke of a key. This knowledge now became available to all SGD groups who in fact began to demand it be revealed.

The second bomb that dislodged the heteronormative exclusivity was that client groups started to hold doctors, therapists, academics and the law accountable. Armed with knowledge as power, SGD group members began to determine their own fate by pressuring changes to treatment policies and laws to afford SGD groups more equal civil rights. It is still a battle that rages today but many years later, it is far more advanced throughout the world and is continuing.

The move to create new family structures is under constant revolution and reinvention. Single parenting has become so common that many people are not waiting to be accepted by others in order to create families. People from SGD groups are finding new ways to form families with and without partners.

The biological and social sciences are often obsessed with establishing norms and certainly for research purposes baselines are needed to compare deviations from the norm. The ideal baseline is static and constant to allow those comparatives to be valid. Norms, however, are relative to the point of observation. Most people believe that their beliefs, opinions and way of living should be the norm. Since being from an SGD group is not and never will be the norm, people from these groups are constantly bombarded by assaults on their existence by an array of individuals and parties.

This means that people from SGD groups live exposed to a constant barrage of attacks, as can be seen in this text, from many different directions in their lives. Not only are these attacks on a personal level, but they are also on a social level via the media colouring how the public see them.

In 2019 in Germany, clergy at the Commission for Marriage and Family of the German Bishops' Conference declared homosexuality a "normal form of sexual predisposition" (Milton, 2019). This meant that there could be no ethical objection to SGD groups in the church. This falls in line with central European human rights policies.

However, Germany, a country known for sexual tolerance, is seeing a resurgence of the far-right, with a greater number of Alternative for Germany (AfG) politicians getting elected, which is worrying and signals it is in danger of fading back to Nazi policies (Eddy, 2017).

Meanwhile, Polish bishops, while saying people from LGBTIQ+ groups deserve respect, said these groups were aiming to "force moral and cultural transformation by gradually accustoming society to behaviours that until recently were considered morally reprehensible" (Polish Bishops Call For Clinics to Help LGBT People, 2020). The bishops also called for clinics to help people revert to what they described as their "natural" sexual orientation, meaning going into conversion therapy to reinstate them towards a supposed heterosexuality. This is a clear attempt to erase LGBTIQ+ groups. Even though Poland is in the European Union, it is moving closer towards the current homophobic and transphobic attitudes of the Russian government under Putin.

These social pressures on SGD people throughout the world, and at times the fear of violence, can lead many people's default mental state to be wariness and alarm. When you are constantly having to dodge bullets in life, you remain in a state of alarm for longer and that becomes your norm.

However, as psychiatry and psychology have lost control of pathologising a state of sex and/or gender diversity, and control of those people's life decisions, they have now shifted towards trying to identify what they perceive to be fundamental mental faults in these groups. A study across five datasets found that transgender and gender-diverse individuals were 3.03 to 6.36 times more likely to be autistic compared to the rest of the population (Warrier et al., 2020).

It is clear from the biological studies I have quoted that there are genetic and developmental differences for many gender diverse people, but not all. These, however, relate to sex development that affects mental perception. But the above autism study in transgender people, and many autism studies in general, over-diagnose due to over-extension of the criteria observed. This implies that self-perceptions of gender diversity may be linked to autistic mental neurodevelopment diversity, which is absurd.

Here we have more desperate attacks by medicine and science on the natural occurrence of sex and/or gender diversity. Again, these attempts to try to find mental problems in intersex and trans people are intersex- and transphobic. It is looking for people from SGD groups' wrongness the moment they walk through the clinic door for help and is a bourgeois attempt to wrestle back control over their lives. Yes, there are people from SGD groups who will have problems related to autism, and sometimes gifts, and it is important to acknowledge them, but to start a clinical assessment with that presumption is oppressive.

The mental health difficulties that many people from SGD groups experience are not necessarily the results of neurodevelopmental faults but instead due to social oppression, ostracisation, threats of violence and loss of human rights, constantly pushing us into the fight or flight response far more than the average person. For many, it is in actual fact our norm. Every time we turn on the news or read the media, we are faced with daily stories of attacks upon our community.

Education has been changing in a piecemeal fashion with a stream of occasional political regressions for people from SGD groups. Middle-class and upper-class members of SGD groups have always been partly protected by wealth and privilege with regards to education. This meant they could often attain a level of adult professionalism that allowed them to make a living and at times live comfortably.

For the average SGD child or adult from a working-class or poor background, however, education is still patchy at times depending on the country, areas and political landscape in which they live. Poor acceptance has forced many of those children and people out of education due to discrimination and minority stress so they were unable to do well within the workforce. Here we see historical factors compounded by discrimination to produce a snowball effect that ripples throughout the person's life.

Many intersex and trans people have passed through their lives stealth without the public knowing about their differences. Consequently, they enjoy heteronormative privilege and do not encounter the aforementioned levels of disadvantage.

When it has become known publicly, however, that a child or adult in education is from a SGD group they can face discrimination, rejection and disadvantage, particularly in publicly-funded education. Here the research is poor and often conflated with LGBTIQ+ research, which distorts the picture so we are left with evidence from individual cases.

Many people living as males from SGD groups become stealth and pass as males, avoiding that educational bias and discrimination. In most countries, there are nearly always more publicly-identified trans females than trans males. Also living and passing as male gives a great educational, social and economic advantage in all countries in the world at present due to the patriarchal social structures.

Those intersex and trans children and people living as female encounter double discrimination due to male privilege and female disadvantages in society, particularly in cultures where females have less social value and fewer human rights. Gaining accolades and achievements in education may not necessarily produce any advantage in male-dominated societies.

The root of disadvantage or social mobility in an industrialised society generally comes back to the level of education. Societies reward scholars and generally try to restrict difference. For the large part, education is geared towards training a person to fit into the commercial world.

With the emergence of children being publicly identified as coming from SGD groups, greater accommodation within the educational systems is now keeping more of those children in education. It follows through that more are going onto higher education and into professions that allow them to become more socially affluent.

We can see, for example, the Australian state of Victoria's educational policy for intersex, trans and gender diverse children's right to education without harassment (Victorian State Government, 2020). Tertiary institutions like the University of Edinburgh in Scotland have also brought in equal rights policies for SGD groups with frequent changes driven by student unions, but at times opposed by conservative or extreme religious student groups (University of Edinburgh, 2020).

Anti-discrimination laws, re-thinking of educational policies and protection for those children and people from SGD groups have contributed to this forward movement. However, due to the upswing of extreme right-wing politics, since the Global Economic Crisis in 2008, subsequent global recession and exclusions by right-wing governments that slipped into law during COVID-19 lockdowns, SGD groups' advances in education at times have met resistance. Overall, however, they are improving piece by piece en masse.

We see that many trans and intersex people living as female and occasionally some living as male from SGD groups enter the sex industry in order to make a living, pay for medical treatment and at times simply to survive in a society that is frequently hostile towards them (Nadal et al., 2013). This still continues in many countries today including South America, Britain, the USA, European countries, Thailand, India, Pakistan and more. This further marginalises SGD groups in society and increases minority stress.

It also exposes them to greater harassment from law enforcement agencies as many work as street sex workers. Added to that can be the burden of racism, particularly in the US, where African American and LatinX sex workers report they are more likely to receive harassment from the police than their Caucasian counterparts (Harper Jean Tobin National Center for Transgender Equality, 2015).

Since sex workers are frequently demonised and marginalised, they tend to live on the margins of society and may not be eligible for social welfare payments or healthcare benefits. Some may have problems finding business, meaning they are living a hard, hand-to-mouth existence: homeless, uneducated, racially discriminated against and unable to afford hormones or surgery. Those layered levels of stress for an extended period makes them vulnerable to drug and alcohol use, mental illness, high-risk or unsafe sexual activities, physical health problems and a shorter life expectancy.

When those identified intersex and trans women present at homeless shelters, often run by religious organisations, they can be turned away and told they are not real women, adding insult to injury. Such organisations use the excuse of protecting vulnerable women from possible male aggression or rape but in reality they are operating their own intersexphobic and transphobic prejudices.

Chantell Martin described how as a trans woman she was turned away from a Sydney women's homeless shelter for being transgender (Sainty, 2015). After the collapse of her relationship, she lost her home, couch surfed and then lived in her car. Being in a women's homeless shelter was an access point for moving toward qualifying for social housing. Sending her to a men's homeless shelter would leave her vulnerable to violence and rape. This kind of rejection of an intersex or trans woman, through barring them from women's homeless shelters in Sydney and other places, is common.

We can see how the Trump administration encouraged Housing and Urban Development rules for homeless shelters to permit the rejection of women whom they suspect of being intersex or trans (Burns, 2020). Unqualified staff would be able to say things like, "You're too tall, masculine, have a deep voice and you are not feminine enough for us to give you shelter."

The acceptability of differing aesthetics has also been changing in many parts of the world. When the transsexual British *Vogue* model April Ashley was outed in the newspapers in the 1960s, all of her modelling contracts and work dried up (Ashley, 2006). Besieged by the gutter press, she spent years trying to outlive her infamy and was assaulted in the street at times. While she was considered beautiful, the fashion industry rejected her and she was relegated to public freak status. Tracie Norman, the African American model who was the face of Clairol Hair Color in the 1970s, had the doors of the American fashion industry slammed in her face when she was outed as a trans woman in 1980 (Yuan and Wong, 2020).

Today fashion houses seek out models who are intersex like Hanne Gaby Odiele (Time, 2017) and trans women like Andreja Pejić (Entertainment Tonight, 2014). Both fitted into the fashion world as it went through an androgynous stage. They both have had highly successful careers as women.

The Actress Laverne Cox broke barriers by being the first known African American and openly trans actress to be nominated for an Emmy award for her work on the Netflix show *Orange is the New Black* (Gjorgievska, 2014). Chaz Bono, a trans man and offspring of the recording artist Cher, has appeared on several TV shows. The trans male comedian and actor Ian Harvie has also appeared in television shows (Whitney, 2017).

At the moment, more trans people are playing trans roles on the screen, but crossing over into playing cis roles is still in its infancy. Amanda Saenz, an intersex person, played an intersex character on the TV show *Faking It* (InterACT, 2016a), but at the time of writing, many intersex people in entertainment are still not coming out as intersex. Gender-neutral and androgynous people are generally on the outside fringe and in specialist art movies not on general release. So, entertainment's interest in SGD issues is still generally restricted to queer culture appeal.

Casting directors are afraid that casting a known person from an SGD group as a cis character in a show or film runs the risk of the character not being believed, which distracts from the story and risks a production failure (Perraudin, 2019). It is the kind of prejudice that used to exist around preventing people of colour getting main roles, or having known gay men play heteronormative men. The prejudice is both overt and covert as casting directors never have to explain themselves.

With the advent of progressive TV shows and people from SGD groups posting on social media, there is a greater awareness of these groups in fashion and entertainment, introducing the public to their presence. Many people are less shocked by seeing people who do not exactly fit the sex and gender stereotypes of male and female, particularly young people. Young people can have more political awareness of the valuing of intersex and trans people, as well as other SGD groups being equal in society.

However, this does not necessarily filter through much to some in society who may have a poor education and live in the heteronormative suburbs or microcultures that still see people who are sex and gender different as against nature and unnatural. We can see in places like Texas, where sex education and political education can be low in much of the populous, that people take to the streets at anti-trans rallies and fail to understand even the basic fundamentals of being intersex (Dickson, 2020). In these spaces, people from SGD groups can still experience prejudice, harassment, ostracisation and violence. In these cultures, looking and being the so-called "normal" is still prized as a pass to go through those cultures unimpeded.

Financial freedom is one of the life keys to being beholden to no one. When you have financial freedom, you can make whatever choices you want in life, even living where you want.

You can place yourself in an environment that supports you, not denigrates you. People who are different, like those from SGD groups, can be shut out of the industrial system so their ability to make money is constricted, except for a few very smart entrepreneurs. The majority of SGD groups have often been and are ostracised in society so they were unable to build wealth. Many live and grow old in poverty.

This has been changing; as more and more people from SGD groups come out in public, it adds to the normalising effect. Societies, by the sheer weight and volume of identified out sex and gender diverse people, can become more accepting and give more opportunities to those minorities. It becomes a ripple effect, helping those minorities climb from poverty to the middle class.

This is very important in political evolution as the middle class spend money on promoting their own self-interest. Revolution is always scary to the public and destabilising to the social order; so most societies generally choose the evolution of human rights, which has been and is happening for SGD groups, sometimes slowly but persistently progressive.

Those middle-class professionals from SGD groups have been building a public history of being scientists, IT developers, accountants, doctors, therapists, academics, teachers, public servants, soldiers, industrialists, writers, filmmakers, entertainers, movie stars, politicians and business owners. They not only have money to influence and lobby for social change, but they also influence through having a high public profile, contacts and knowing how to work the system.

Family is the heart of all societies and their needs are the central core of any election campaign as politicians play to the needs and fears of the family unit. The worst thing a politician can ever do is attack the family unit, which is why politicians have spent so much time being photographed kissing babies on the campaign trail.

What they are saying is, "We are just like you, the majority of society, so vote for us and you vote for yourself", and the public swallow that propaganda. The public vote just as they shop: emotionally, not logically. Plying the public with intellect and common sense always fails in politics but playing to their emotions could get the dead elected to office.

This social landscape changes as more people from SGD groups are being seen in public with their families like the actor Warren Beatty's son Stephen. That makes it harder for extreme right-wing fascists to engage in character assassination of those people because they would also be seen as attacking their families, which could backfire. While many people from families of choice live with intersex and trans and gender diverse people, it does not presently demand the same media headline as a biological relative of a famous person connected to someone from a SGD group.

You can tell an adult you think they are the devil and they should die, but when you publicly tell a parent their child is evil, you step over a well-recognised unacceptable social boundary. You become a child abuser, attacking the family unit. Many voters will not maintain their support for those politicians who are seen to be attacking those families and even right-wing voters may abandon them.

There is, however, a disconnect at the moment with intersex people as few publicly identified intersex people are seen in the media with their families. If surgery was performed on a child, without their permission, those people can often feel deceived by their doctors and birth families, which causes family splits. Older public intersex figures like Georgina Somerset, Dawn Langley-Simmons and Lady Colin-Campbell all understood the power of the publicity of being seen with families, but many of today's campaigners for intersex equal rights have yet to fully embrace this strategy.

Trans woman Caitlyn Jenner received a lot of support in

American society when she transitioned because she was surrounded by her family. Later, however, on the release of her memoir, *The Secrets of My Life* (Jenner, 2017), public reports emerged of splits within the family about the contents of the book. It was perhaps not the best PR move on Jenner's part and possibly lost her some public support (Aiello, 2018).

Chaz Bono, however, gained great public support when he transitioned to male, in part because of the close bond between him and his mother, the singer and actress Cher. While she initially struggled with his transition, she soon became very publicly supportive, which has made his transition in public life much easier and the public more accepting of his transition (Shannon, 2018). Any publicist will teach you that if you are in disfavour in the public eye, get yourself photographed with your family to restore your wholesome image.

There have now been many people from SGD groups who have become public in local and national politics. Tony Briffa, an intersex person, became the Mayor of the Council of Hobsons Bay in Australia in 2009 (Intersex Human Rights Australia, 2017). A trans woman, Georgina Beyer, was elected Mayor of Carterton in 1995 in New Zealand and then to the New Zealand Parliament in 2002 but did not stand again for the 2005 elections (New Zealand Parliament, 2019). Vladimir Luxuria was a trans woman who served in the European Parliament from 2006 to 2008 (Shoffman, 2006), while Joanne Marie Conte, who transitioned to become a trans woman, was elected to the Arvada City Council, USA, in 1991 (Martin, 2013). Petra De Sutter was elected the Deputy Prime Minister of Belgium in 2020 (Woodyatt & Frater, 2020). The list could continue right up to today.

Politics is all about personality and appealing to the public mentality of the moment, the issues people are worried about and what they want to experience in their daily life. It seems there are no barriers to people from SGD groups getting into politics in many parts of the world if their legal status is legitimate and at times, even if it is not.

It is such a precarious profession, however, and many elected officials are lucky to last more than a few terms. Other politicians will go to extraordinary lengths to oust their opponent by concocting campaigns to denigrate the person from the SGD group in public, so it is not for the faint-hearted. Greater civil rights have been growing due to those who have served, not only through their direct action and lobbying, but also through working the contacts they made during their service.

There have been great improvements in the world for many people from SGD groups; however, this is not true for all of them. Political influence, extreme religious views, family disharmony, ignorance and social unrest still leave many SGD groups in many parts of the world with little expectation of quality of life, often making suicide seem a better option.

Oppression operates on many levels for people from SGD groups. Legal discrimination can leave many without the proper documents to match their identity. This leaves many living their lives precariously in the shadows for fear of being singled out, attacked and abused. The lack of the right to be yourself legally places you as an outlaw in the culture in which you were born. You are cast as a pariah and outcast.

The sheer lack of legal protection against this oppression causes people from a SGD group to feel very insecure and frequently in a constant state of anxiety. When the laws do not offer those protections, the public always abuses their power to oppress. The lack of legal protection by society is blatantly macro-oppression that is legalised omission of human rights when discrimination is sanctioned by society at large.

Just because you may be able to exist in places where laws legally protect you, does not mean that the laws also protect you against covert oppression and discrimination. Covert is as pernicious as overt oppression; it may be silent, but it is equally as deadly. Covert micro-oppression within small groups and sub-cultures is less obvious to the law. It is guarded by the right of freedom of speech and the ability to gather while excluding others who might not share your faith or philosophy. While there are the legitimate rights of specialist groups to gather, they can be breeding grounds for shunning people who are different from them including SGD groups, denying the latter's very existence.

Extreme right-wing groups and religious zealots will always demonise the image of someone who is other than strictly male or female as being wrong, feeding that paranoia and hate out into their communities and groups. While idealistically being from a SGD group in families and society would be easier if it were more normalised, this is a long way off because SGD groups are such a small part of the human race and tribalism favours the majority. They will always be outliers, different and at times rejected, harassed and experience minority stress, which for many will lead to thoughts, feelings and actions that will initiate suicide.

References

Aiello, M. (2018). Caitlyn Jenner says it's "tought" to maintain a "close" bond with her family. *ENews*. Retrieved from https://www.eonline.com/news/938119/caitlyn-jenner-says-it-s-tough-to-maintain-a-close-bond-with-her-family

Ashley, A. (2006). *The first lady*. John Black.

Burns, K. (2020). The Trump administration's proposed homeless shelter rule spells out how to spot a trans woman: The Housing and Urban Development proposal instructs shelters to try to identify trans women by height, facial hair, and Adam's apples. *Vox*. Retrieved from https://www.vox.com/

identities/2020/7/17/21328708/proposed-anti-trans-rule-homeless-shelters-judge-women

Campbell, L.C. (1997). *A life worth living.* Little, Brown and Company.

Council of Europe. (2015). Human Rights and Intersex People (1st ed). Retrieved from https://rm.coe.int/16806da5d4

Dickson, E. (2020). How a Texas custody case became a terrifying right-wing talking point. *Rolling Stone.* Retrieved from https://www.rollingstone.com/culture/culture-features/transgender-custody-case-dallas-anne-georgulas-mark-younger-904433/

Eddy, M. (2017, September 25). Alternative for Germany: Who are they, and what do they want? *The New York Times.* Retrieved from https://www.nytimes.com/2017/09/25/world/europe/germany-election-afd.html

Entertainment Tonight. (2014). Meet the world's most successful transgender model. Retrieved from https://www.youtube.com/watch?v=kcymKf5X0LQ

Harper Jean Tobin National Center for Transgender Equality (2015). Meaningful work: Transgender experiences in the sex trade. *National Center for Transgender Equality.* Retrieved from https://transequality.org/sites/default/files/Meaningful%20Work-Full%20Report_FINAL_3.pdf

Gizauskas, R. (2019, February 15). 'I FELT SHAME' I am a girl but aged 16 doctors told me I was 'genetically a BOY' – and being intersex means I have more love to give in relationships. *The Sun.* Retrieved from https://www.thesun.co.uk/fabulous/8420077/intersex-woman-suicidal-cancer-battle-suz-temko/

Gjorgievska, A. & Rothman, L. (2014). Laverne Cox is the first transgender person nominated for an Emmy —

She explains why that matters. *Time.* Retrieved from http://time.com/2973497/laverne-cox-emmy/

InterACT. (2016a). Live hangout with Amanda Saenz and Emily Quinn. Retrieved from https://www.youtube.com/watch?v=V4jgkYEDPN4

InterACT. (2016b). Statement on intersex terminology. Retrieved from https://interactadvocates.org/interact-statement-on-intersex-terminology/

Intersex Human Rights Australia. (2017, October 26). Tony Briffa: My experience as the first openly intersex mayor. Retrieved from https://ihra.org.au/10543/briffa-first-intersex-mayor/

Jenner, C. (2017). *The secrets of my life* (1st ed). Grand Central Publishing

Langley-Simmons, D. (1995). *Dawn: A Charleston legend.* Wyrick & Company

Man who won '66 women's downhill gives up medal. (2015, February 3). *Los Angeles Times.* Retrieved from www.latimes.com/archives/la-xpm-1988-11-19-sp-422-story

Martin, C. (2013, February). Joanne Conte's life story a complex tale of gender, politics. *The Denver Post.* Retrieved from https://www.denverpost.com/2013/02/02/joanne-contes-life-story-a-complex-tale-of-gender-politics/

Meyer, W., Bockting, W., Cohen-Kettenis, P., Coleman, E., Diceglie, D., Devor, H., Gooren, L., Joris, J., Kirk, S., Kuiper, B., Laub, D., Lawrence, A., Menard, Y., Patton, J., Schaefer, L., Webb, A. & Wheeler, C. (2002). The Harry Benjamin International Gender Dysphoria Association's Standards of Care. *United Journal of Psychology & Human Sexuality,* 13(1), 1-30. Retrieved from https://doi.org/10.1300/J056v13n01_01

Milton, J. (2019). German bishops declare that homosexuality is completely and utterly 'normal'. *PinkNews*. Retrieved from https://www.pinknews.co.uk/2019/12/14/german-bishops-homosexuality-normal-berlin/

Nadal, K., Davidoff, K. & Fujii-Doe, K. (2013). Transgender women and the sex work industry: Roots in systemic, institutional, and interpersonal discrimination. *Journal of Trauma & Dissociation*, 5(2). Retrieved from https://www.tandfonline.com/doi/abs/10.1080/15299732.2014.867572

New Zealand Parliament (2019). Beyer, Georgina. Retrieved from https://www.parliament.nz/en/mps-and-electorates/former-members-of-parliament/beyer-georgina/

Perraudin, F., (2019). Cast more transgender actors in non-trans roles, union urges. *The Guardian*. Retrieved from www.theguardian.com/society/2019/oct/28/cast-more-transgender-actors-in-non-trans-roles-union-urges

Polish bishops call for "clinics to help LGBT people regain natural sexual orientation". (2020). *Notes From Poland*. Retrieved from https://notesfrompoland.com/2020/08/30/polish-bishops-call-for-clinics-to-help-lgbt-people-regain-natural-sexual-orientation/

Sainty, L. (2015). Transgender women are falling through cracks in Australia's homeless system. *Buzzfeed*. Retrieved from https://www.buzzfeed.com/lanesainty/transgender-women-are-falling-through-cracks-in-australias-h

Shannon, M. (2018, September 2). The complex family history of Cher's kids, Chaz Bono and Elijah Allman. *Monagiza*. Retrieved from http://www.monagiza.com/stories/complex-family-history-chers-kids-chaz-bono-elijah-allman/

Shoffman, M. (2006, April 19). Italy elects Europe's first transgender MP. *PinkNews*. Retrieved from https://www.pinknews.co.uk/2006/04/19/italy-elects-europes-first-transgender-mp/

The EU Parliament's LGBTI Intergroup & Children's Rights Intergroup. (2019, February 14). Urgent need to address intersex human rights violations, says European Parliament. Retrieved from https://lgbti-ep.eu/2019/02/14/urgent-need-to-address-intersex-human-rights-violations-says-european-parliament/

Time (2017). Hanne Gaby Odiele on modelling career & being an intersex activist. Retrieved from https://www.youtube.com/watch?v=mz_05iJI31U

Turtle, G. (1963). *Over the sex border.* Victor Gollancz Ltd.

University of Edinburgh. (2010). *Trans equality policy.* Retrieved from https://www.ed.ac.uk/files/atoms/files/trans_equality_policy.pdf

Victorian State Government. (2020). *School policy, gender identity.* Retrieved from https://www.education.vic.gov.au/school/principals/spag/health/Pages/genderidentity.aspx

Warrier, V., Greenberg, D., Weir, E., Buckingham, C., Smith, P., Meng-Chuan. L., Allison, C. & Baron-Cohen, S. (2020). Elevated rates of autism, other neurodevelopmental and psychiatric diagnoses, and autistic traits in transgender and gender-diverse individuals. *Nature Communications.* Retrieved from https://www.nature.com/articles/s41467-020-17794-1

Whitney, E.O. (2019). Meet Ian Harvie, the 'transparent' actor playing the authentic trans roles he never got to see on screen. *Screen Crush.* Retrieved from https://screencrush.com/ian-harvie-interview-our-hollywood/

Woodyatt, A. & Frater, J. (2020, October 2). Belgium's new Deputy Prime Minister is Europe's most senior transgender politician. *CNN*. Retrieved from https://edition.cnn.com/2020/10/02/europe/belgium-deputy-pm-de-sutter-intl-scli/index.html

Yuan, J. & Wong, A. (2020). The first black trans model had her face on a box of Clairol. *The Cut*. Retrieved from https://www.thecut.com/2015/12/tracey-africa-transgender-model-c-v-r.html

Chapter 9:
Provision of Care

The delivery of care for mental health patients and the delivery of services, suicide prevention and care for sex and/or gender diverse (SDG) groups differ vastly throughout the world. Some countries have high levels of care while others have little or no care at all. The influences that affect that delivery are political, religious, social, economic and locational. Achieving best practice for these groups can be difficult at times as healthcare services are often at the mercy of politics.

Sectioning Individuals With Sex or Gender Suicidation
The hospitalisation model of suicide intervention has very mixed results in the general population and is not generally useful in treating people from SGD groups unless they have a severe mental illness. Detaining someone from a SGD group at risk of suicide and locking them up in a secure psychiatric unit for assessment over 48 hours may not treat their situation or erase minority stress. In fact, in many cases, it can increase their sense of being wrong and determination to suicide.

It may also increase resistance to treatment rather than open rapport for immediate intervention. Health professionals treating suicidation for people from SGD groups need to advocate on the clients' behalf to keep them in the community as much as possible with emergency support.

Psychiatric assessment and testing of SGD groups are constantly subject to operator, situational, interpretation and cultural distortion. The historical zeitgeist of pathologisation of these groups by psychiatry weighs heavily on the shoulders of SGD groups. It is evident that a diagnosis of mental illness can ignore the familial, social and cultural displacement that leads to SGD minority stress.

Clients in this situation can be given a whole host of misdiagnosis labels prejudiced from the psychiatric gestalt, medicated and then live out the diagnosis. They can be institutionalised, become long-term social welfare dependents and locked into the psychiatric system, continuing to deteriorate mentally and emotionally. The medications may switch off their fight and flight response initially but their cognitive reasoning may never evolve beyond the trauma. The suicidal thoughts can remain long-term as the person is depressed, dysfunctional, dependent and often carries out suicide by some means later in their life.

In Perth, Australia the local mental health services declared a code yellow in October 2018 (Cross, 2018). David Mountain, the Chair of the Faculty of the Australasian College of Emergency Medicine, commented that there were not enough emergency bed spaces so a code yellow was often declared. Some emergency mental health patients have to spend days in the emergency wards until a placement becomes available. Perth is one of the remotest cities in the world and has a chronic shortage of nurses and mental health staff, yet it is in a rich country.

In 2019, an Australian Productivity Commission report stated that the care shortage problem was endemic across Australia and unfortunately, some of those unattended patients do manage to carry out suicide while waiting for appropriate ward places (Australasian College of Emergency Medicine, 2019). The report also found that up to one-third of emergency mental health patients, after being discharged, had no follow-up contact with mental health services after seven days.

Principles of Provision

When managers and policymakers create services and allocate funds for helping people from SGD groups, decisions, policies, processes, procedures, protocols and practices need to be run through an ethical inventory. This process also needs to be the same for healthcare practitioners and practitioner cross-referrals.

Does the service you offer or refer on to meet ethics standards for the care of SGD groups of people?

This is important to consider because most services provided by state and private bodies in many countries or regions currently do not meet ethical standards. As you will see from this book, intergenerational trauma exists for people from SGD groups because of the poor-quality, unethical care they have encountered in the past, frequently without their permission or against their will.

Mani Bruce (Lahood, 2012) talks about how they underwent unnecessary surgery to their genitals as an intersex child in order to give them a stereotypical female appearance. This robbed Bruce of much of the ability to enjoy sexual pleasure, and they believe it was a major cause of them being unable to maintain a loving relationship during adulthood. Thousands of other people are now stepping forward with similar stories.

Lady Colin-Campbell (1997) wrote about how after being born intersex and wishing to be treated as a girl, she had to endure the forced administration of testosterone therapy as a teenager, which masculinised her in ways she did not want. Her father conspired with a medical practitioner to force the treatment upon her because he thought she should be living as male, ignoring her wishes.

This practice of attempting to cosmetically normalise intersex children's genitalia to resemble male or female, when there is no immediate medical danger, is based on intersexphobia by cis heteronormative people. It was devised by the practices at Johns Hopkins Hospital in America and based on the ideas, propagated by the psychologist John Money (1996). He proposed that a child could be raised and convinced to be the sex and gender they are told they are.

This practice of trying to train a child to be a gender has proved to have failed in many cases. Most notably, in the case of David Reimer who suffered a circumcision accident, then he was raised as girl, and eventually completed suicide (Colapinto, 2000). No funding should be provided to healthcare services that still support this model.

April Ashley (2006) tells how she was subject to electric shock treatment in the 1950s as a teenager because she identified as being transsexual. At that time, transsexualism was considered by her treating clinicians to be a mental illness and delusion. A whole generation of people were treated as delusional and suffering from sexual perversion simply because they were sex or gender diverse. In many parts of the world today, this is still the case.

Professor Deirdre McCloskey (1999), an American economics academic, wrote about how her own sister, a mental health professional, took action to have her compulsorily detained in an emergency psychiatric unit for observation when she announced she was transitioning from male to female. The assumption by many health professionals that the desire to transition to another sex or gender is some kind of dreaded delusional state is common, even today.

Norrie May-Welby who won the right in the High Court of Australia (2014) to have their documents state that they were 'sex non-specific' found that many years later the Australian Medicare system was still refusing, illegally, to have any other options on Medicare records than male or female.

Christie Elan-Cane (Blackstone Chambers, 2018) in the UK fought for over 20 years to have an X on their passport, in accordance with international civil aviation guidelines. Elan-Cane took their fight all the way to the UK's High Court. They identify as neither male nor female.

The treatment of people from SGD groups generally lacks input from those groups and individuals themselves. This bourgeoisie heteronormative approach has been to treat such people as delusional rather than consulting with them to find out what help they need. It is a top-down approach to medicine and ignores the social contract between members of society to respect self-autonomy.

Intergenerational trauma is a reality in these groups of people who frequently, over the past 150 years, have been legally, socially and medically abused and still are abused throughout the world today. The offences against them have frequently been buried, hidden, erased and not publicly acknowledged or discussed.

That intergenerational abuse has led to enforced medical treatments, denial of medical treatment, social and economic disadvantage, harassment, prejudice, bullying, political persecution, depression, suicide and frequently murder. This is still continually happening today and is likely to continue due to minority victimisation.

So, when people from these groups come into contact with healthcare workers, they can bring with them that sense and history of intergenerational SGD trauma as well as their personal traumas. They will very possibly carry with them the fear of being judged and of being treated unfairly. It is paramount that organisations offer sensitivity trainings to all healthcare professionals helping these groups and ensure their staff are aware and educated about their histories.

A study of transgender and gender diverse health and wellbeing, published by the Department of Health, Victoria in Australia (2014), in coordination with Latrobe University, reported that many trans and intersex people experienced extreme prejudice when accessing health services.

More disturbing was the fact that people were mocked and refused service simply because they were from SGD groups. The absolute irony of the study was that the title of the study itself was prejudicial by using the word 'transgender' when talking about the interests of multiple SGD groups of people.

All funding and services need to incorporate these policies:
1. Intersex children, children and adults with sex anomalies, who are in no medical danger, should not be subject to surgery or medical intervention without their informed consent, with their options fully explained to them.
2. Intersex children and children with sex anomalies should be able to elect to have surgeries and medical intervention at any medically safe time, when they acquire cognitive reasoning and understand risk analysis.
3. Children and adults who developed cross-sex identification from how their sex was registered at birth, should have an age-appropriate right to medical intervention to affirm that sex and gender.
4. All records should have the option for a person to elect a third identification other than male or female, without having to specifically indicate what that might be, e.g. X or non-specific.
5. All healthcare services providing specifically for SGD groups of people should partake in community consultation on policies with those groups as stakeholders, whether those service providers are government bodies or community interest groups.
6. All public healthcare services providing specifically for SGD groups of people should have members from those groups on their governing board to guide the organisation.
7. All public healthcare services providing specifically for SGD groups of people should have people from those

groups on their staff.

8. The provision of care and funding to SGD groups of people should be equally prioritised along with equivalent health services.

9. All public services for SGD groups of people should actively publish any discriminatory practices publicly.

10. Any publicly funded organisation that engages in discriminatory practices against SGD groups of people should undergo a review and re-education programs. They should have funding withdrawn if the reorientation does not result in the organisation adopting anti-discriminatory practices.

11. Any practitioner who engages in discriminatory practices against SGD groups of people, in or out of the workplace, should undergo investigation, supervision and review. Persistent offences should culminate in termination of employment and registration.

12. All public organisations providing services for SGD groups of people should invite client feedback and evaluation of the service provided.

13. All health professionals must publicly publish any prejudice they might hold, religious or moral.

14. No person who works for any organisation that receives public funding may refuse service to any person from any SGD group.

Where does the money come from?

When people are on the brink of suicide, they are frequently poor, although this is not necessarily always the case. Certainly, lower socioeconomic groups are traditionally less able to access the level of treatment they may need to improve their physical and mental health. Healthcare, after all, costs money and not every government provides a cradle to grave healthcare service.

If you have money, you can shop around for the private care you believe you need. If you are poor or on a low income, you generally have to avail yourself of the health services provided by the government or a charity. Such services may be minimal, offering lower clinical hours, are not as in-depth or do not offer the facilities that private care is able to.

Private facilities may also have the extra added bonus of clients being able to offset some of the costs against their private health insurance. However, that can at times require a psychopathological diagnosis.

What drives national and regional provision, low provision, withdrawal and denial of care are local and national politics. These politics control funding but they also control policy reliant on decisions based on voting numbers, electoral promises and the manipulation of political public relations.

Interlaced into this are the prejudices and morals of the majority government politicians of the day. Ministerial interference in the status quo can create legacies they wish to leave from their time in office. It frequently savages the provision of care of minorities who are generally not seen politically as substantial voters. This particularly happens when it comes to SGD groups, as they are frequently positioned as a low-impact voting group, anti-social or groups who are drains on society's resources.

Bach (2018) reported how the US Trump administration sought to roll back the Obama era protection of transgender people. The major initiator, the Department of Health and Human Services, was proposing that people could only be identified according to their original recorded or diagnosed biological sex, which would be strictly male or female. If and when such policies were implemented, it would have not only made many, if not all, people from SGD groups illegitimate, but would also have caused a massive withdrawal of government-funded health services and affected the ability of private health funds to give rebates for treatments.

The dramatic national change in political health service policies between the supportive Obama pro-SGD groups era and the Trump anti-SGD groups era occurred within two years. It shows how tenuous health services for all SGD groups can be as the political pendulum swings, which can happen in any country in a short period. This kind of policy change can also happen on a regional level in local politics.

Local politics are more concerned with funding rivalry between service providers and funding within organisations. Funding is generally allocated by two methods. Firstly, on disease prevention-based policies like treatment of HIV, sexually transmitted diseases or cancer care services and so on. The higher the epidemiological statistics for disease transmission and occurrence, the higher the political agenda and the more funds become available.

Many organisations throughout the world have tacked services for SGD groups onto their services funded directly or indirectly, wholly or partly through sexually transmitted disease funding, including suicide prevention, including ACON (ACON, Council of NSW, 2020), Australia; The Center New York, USA (2020); and the Los Angeles LGBT Center, USA (2020). Some organisations like QMUNITY (2020) in Canada seek multiple sources of funding and grants in order to offer low-cost counselling.

Some of these facilities are also funded with funds from the second kind of funding, which goes directly to SGD groups or involves redirected funds from queer organisations or funding. They can receive national grants and local funding according to the politics of the day and region. Services can be specifically for SGD groups or within facilities for LGBTIQ+ services. As always, provision of funds are not guaranteed and can be tenuous at all times from year to year.

The services may be centred at particular static locations within a city or town, and they may also be part of satellite projects with the different services delivered in different places for economic reasons or the locations available for clients. Local politics are important to consider because they determine how clients relate to or have access to those services.

Intersex people tend not to use services directed at the LGBTIQ+ community because those services often do not have the expertise on intersex issues. They may not have the medical or psychological understanding of the issues intersex people face, even though they have claimed funds to service this client group. This means those funds can tend to be swallowed up by that organisation to use for other clients.

Many intersex people will also not use facilities directed at transgender people because they do not want to be thought of as transgender and those staff also tend not to understand their issues. Intersex people tend to use the services of endocrinological and surgical clinics where little or no mental health support is offered, so their suicide issues get relegated to the regular mental health services where they are very rarely understood.

Many trans people can tend not to use many of the services directed at LGBTIQ+ groups either because once again they are frequently faced with staff who do not understand their issues. These organisations may claim to facilitate this client group but frequently do not understand their issues and swallow up the money, leaving people from the SGD groups dealing with suicide issues without the specialist care to which they can relate.

Organisations fight fiercely for funding and will often tack any label they can onto the services they declare they will or do provide to get extra funding, but frequently they do not provide those services for SGD groups. It can be a fight to the death as those organisations can collapse without the funding, but unfortunately it leads to many SGD groups not being properly facilitated.

What also happens is the organisations tend to provide

the wrong care by the wrong staff to most of the clients from SGD groups and those services are not targeted. Organisations often buy in the services of qualified mental health professionals. This is an economic decision as they may bring in funding of their own or they are cheaper than having in-house services, but unfortunately, they often have no specific understanding of the issues of many SGD client groups.

A 22-year-old intersex woman, just having found out she has AIS, may be in shock, questioning her identity and considering suicide because her parents had lied to her. She is unlikely to want to talk to a male gay counsellor who has no idea about AIS. Neither does a trans man renting his body in a sex dungeon to pay for surgery necessarily need advice from a healthcare professional who has no experience of having worked with people like himself. Nor does he want to work with someone who has no idea of the nightly pressures and risks he takes that led him to overdose on heroin.

In creating services for people from SGD groups who are wrestling with suicide, organisations need to get more honest about their real capabilities, and stop taking funding for services they do not and cannot provide because they do not have the expertise. When a person faces suicide, they need to be able to connect with a clinician who has a good understanding of their background and issues and can help them do the work to recover fast and not just lead the client to continue to suffer in survival mode.

One can never expect the average health professional having first contact with someone from a SGD group on the verge of suicide to have in-depth knowledge of the issues the client faces or the remedies that they may be need. As health professionals, we have to deal with a vast array of clients and issues. Therefore, providers' policies must include that those clients from SGD groups can directly and immediately be referred on to specialists in this area and not kept in-house because the client is worth funding to the organisation.

There are intersex and trans clinicians who understand androgyny as well as culturally-specific sex and gender diversity who should be brought into the service so those clients can instantly initiate rapport with them. In cases of suicide, immediate expert help is needed, and the client does not have time for a healthcare worker to negotiate their way around foreign issues. When no local experienced help is available, a remote video link with an outside expert may be a better option.

However, funding is not always available so we run into the issues of finite finances and clients running out of funding allocations, even though the client may need more immediate care. In this case, the client may end up herded into the psychiatric medication model, can be heavily medicated and never deal with their sex and gender issues or suicidal ideation, so they remain heavily medicated and pre-suicidal in the long-term.

When dealing with the provision of care for suicidal people from SGD groups who have additional mental health issues, providers can at times be at a loss as to how to proceed. They may appear in the general psychiatric populations if they have predominantly mental health issues like schizoid personality disorders, borderline or bipolar problems that dominate their care. In extreme cases, it may even be considered that their SGD issues are part of dissociated personality disorders, as an extended alter persona. Expert help on sex and gender issues should, however, still be brought into care plans to assess the levels of risk of suicide from those issues and to either treat or advise on how to treat accordingly. Some of the mental health funding could also be redirected to the client's sex and gender issues.

Online and Electronic Care

The provision of online platforms has become more common although there are ethical confidentiality issues around their use. Platforms are not secure and often belong to and are operated in countries other than the one in which the client lives, so confidentiality is automatically broken. They operate in real-time or delayed time responses and the user often does not know where the responder is or their qualifications. For emergency suicide rescue and prevention, they have limited use when only in the written form as they are too mono-dimensional and the respondent is unable to observe the caller.

Video calls are more informative and interactive and can work well particularly when clients live in remote regions or countries. Legally we again face the issues of electronic confidentiality because of uncontrolled foreign hosting, but it does at least give access to visual observation. These services, however, are more useful for ongoing therapy than emergency suicide prevention unless you are dealing with a deaf client and using sign language.

Telephone suicide rescue lines have a much longer established history. The responder can hear intonations in the voice of the client and elicit real-time responses, which is imperative in suicide rescue. They may also be specialist suicide rescue services and some clients might not want to be seen. It is highly unlikely that the responder will have an in-depth knowledge around sex and gender issues, but they can be very good in dealing with suicidal callers as the responders are trained in suicide prevention and may work with those issues daily.

Electronically-led consumer healthcare is now determining how much remote healthcare is being delivered and will be delivered in future. Many leaders in healthcare management, however, are still working off old healthcare delivery models, which are beginning to become obsolete. Younger people source their information electronically and do not congregate in the ways of older generations. They have astute electronic shopping skills, become very specific in what they are shopping for and are not just random shoppers. The use of meeting apps and social media platforms mean that they are involved in a whole different world from those who are currently at the top of the mental health management tree.

When we look at the websites and online data of service providers, we can see the often extremely poor quality of electronic presentations, information and contact interactiveness with the client base they are seeking to reach. Many no longer display telephone numbers clearly or at all. Most of them look like webpages thrown together by a disinterested relative and are unappealing to younger, more tech-savvy and interactive generations. There is little understanding of the need to market to client groups; instead they often portray the attitude that people should be grateful they get any information at all. Government-funded organisations do not generally value the need to market to the client groups and do not allocate sufficient funds that are needed to reach those people.

If you look around any major city, you will see the closure of gay, lesbian and trans bars and clubs, as people begin to form communities online that they then translate into meetings. When you look at how intersex people meet each other to commune and exchange experiences, it generally begins online where people can be anonymous at first until they become more comfortable talking to others.

People make up their mind in three to five seconds as to whether the owners of a website or social media group can help them. This includes people seeking relief from suicidal thoughts connected with sex and gender issues. Just because you are a government-funded service does not mean you can be lazy with your marketing or not allocate funds to interact with clients electronically.

Nevertheless, it is worth noting that many clients want face-to-face help that gives them a greater sense of connection, being paid attention to and the ability to have human contact.

Facilitating Younger People and Families

Growing up is a daunting task at times. You are supposed to learn and be so many things, often without a roadmap on how to go forward. You are young and really quite unsure if you can achieve the things you and others expect of you. Many parents are supportive and nurturing of their children, helping them to fulfil their possibilities, but many parents in the world are experiencing social and economic pressures and are just trying to survive on a day-to-day basis.

When you add the pressure of your child having issues around their sex and gender, which you do not understand, to the ordinary everyday life pressures, it can be overwhelming for parents and family. They may go into absolute denial and refuse to discuss the issues, be told by clinicians to keep it a secret, be completely ignorant about what they are seeing or angry it is another pressure upon their lives. They are not necessarily bad parents but are out of their comfort zone, knowledge and abilities to cope with the situation.

One of the most useful processes for supporting children from SGD groups is to provide services for the parents and families to help them handle their unique situation, for which they also have no roadmaps. When a child becomes suicidal because of their issues around sex and gender, family services must step in to assess the family's needs, whether they are equipped to handle the situation and what help, if any, social services can offer, with counselling if necessary.

The child has become a child at risk, not because of their sex or gender diversity but because they have become suicidal, so mandatory reporting by any healthcare worker to child services is obligatory. If you practice in an area or country where there are no child services, it would be wise to bring in the help of local medical workers, charities or religious support networks if the family are of a religious persuasion. You must have done your due diligence in advance to ensure that any services you invite in to help the family do not operate any intersex- or transphobic attitudes. You must also consult with the family to work with them; but remember, the safety of the child is your priority.

Funding for Children

Funding for children can often be sourced from a wider range of payees because they are considered more vulnerable than adults, including paediatrics, hospitals, mental health services, psychiatry, extended funding from general medicine family practices, childcare services and charities. This will require those children to be entered into the system, which can carry with it an automatic social services review of the family situation, including the suitability of the child to live in that environment.

Healthcare workers need to make the families and guardians fully aware of possible environment reviews at the beginning of contact to prepare them for those circumstances. The trauma of a sudden social services review of family circumstances could cause distrust of healthcare professionals and damage the care arrangements of the child. Families also need to be made aware that mandatory reporting is automatic for healthcare workers when a child shows up in the system as suicidal.

Disabled People from SGD Groups

Some people from SGD groups may have physical or mental disabilities. This can magnify and add to any minority stress they experience and cause an accumulated stress response. Often this population can become extremely isolated and not have as much access to services.

If people are blind, deaf or need wheelchair access, healthcare workers must check in advance that they are matched with clinicians and facilities that can provide for their needs. Many projects that offer niche services for people from SGD groups are not set up to deal with people with disabilities because they are low-budget and in fairly inaccessible places. When such clients are ill-matched, it adds to their already complex stress levels.

It is, however, possible at times to redirect some of the disability funding resources the clients may have to help them deal with suicidal issues around their sex and gender. This is well worth exploring.

Sex and gender issues are often dismissed and not given the clinical attention needed. This is particularly common when dealing with clients who have lower intellects, Asperger's, Autism or Down Syndrome. Here regular case conferencing with social workers who advocate on the client's behalf is paramount.

Providing Multi-Racial and Cultural Help to SGD Clients

Language, culture and ethnographic experience all offer different perspectives on sex and gender. This is coloured by education, economic status, politics, law and at times the legality of persons in the country in which they are living.

If a person is an illegal immigrant, accessing any health services can be daunting and poses the threat of deportation, so they often go to backstreet doctors to have medical procedures, at times illegally. The client may be desperate for help at the lowest cost possible. However, this often leads to considerable medical complications with the client becoming suicidal when procedures go wrong.

The Guardian (Ramsay, 2017) reported the illegal trade in plastic surgery in Colombia where surgeries left people with deformities. In Australia, a clinic was prosecuted for illegally injecting mainly Chinese-speaking clients with industrial filers and illegally imported drugs that led to death in one case (Potaka, 2018). Many countries cannot keep up with laws around medical procedures so the consumer, particularly foreign-speaking residents, frequently have procedures carried out by unqualified practitioners.

This can leave the client scared, disadvantaged and suicidal, and also often unable to access legitimate medical or mental health services due to language barriers. So, in setting up government-funded clinics, it is important to provide multiple-language access for clients from SGD groups, particularly if they are suicidal.

Racism is real in medical and mental health services throughout the world and even more so if you are from a SGD group. It complicates things because there are economic and social access issues that go along with being a member of a country's minority or oppressed racial groups. Isolation, exclusion and failure to understand or have access to information can lead to extreme depression when someone is dealing with sex and gender issues, to the extent of inducing self-harming and suicidal ideation.

Community Outreach

Outreach tends to work well when it is specific, client-group targeted or educational and noncontroversial. For instance, it works well in disease control and was used extensively during the HIV crisis to reach gay males and people working in the sex industry, which also allowed access for clients to become research participants. Even in the guise of community-based intervention, the control of HIV in the general population has been very successful (Salam et al., 2014). Locational contact was designed to make contact exactly where those at risk could be found. The same approach has been used to target trans people in the sex industry around the risk of sexually transmitted diseases.

It does not work well when the target group is poorly defined and too broad, taking in people or children who may have religious or social objections to hearing the educational message. We can see how an outreach program in Australia for

LGBTIQ+ children (the SAFE Schools anti-bullying program) met with considerable resistance in the education system as parents with religious objections successfully campaigned to have it banned and withdrawn (Haydar, 2017). The audience was too broad for an easy passage of the message into the educational situation.

Outreach around suicide can also be very difficult for healthcare professionals to deliver as it is a highly sensitive issue that frightens people. When you add the issue of potential suicide to SGD groups, naive audiences can become too confused. They may be intimidated by their lack of knowledge and the seriousness of the risk of suicide goes over their heads. So, if as an organisation you were to engage in outreach around suicide and SGD issues, your audience would be very small and likely only interested parties.

In working with suicidal people from SGD groups, it is necessary to provide the client with a list of the 24-hour suicide rescue lines and telephone numbers that they may call in an emergency out of office hours.

Preferencing Cognitive Behaviour Approaches
Clients who have ample financial resources can choose whatever approaches they like to recover from suicidal thoughts and behaviours. Government projects, not-for-profits and charities, however, do not have the luxury of copious funding. They must stretch the dollar to facilitate as many clients as possible as effectively as they can. The need is for behavioural change as soon as possible for the client to satisfy fund allocation managers. A project that cannot show cost benefit effectiveness will not be able to compete in the funding marketplace.

Brief cognitive behavioural therapy (Bryan & Rudd, 2018) suicide prevention is more acceptable to funders. It can be measured better than other therapies because of its discrete, measured, staged and recorded processes. It can, by its interventionalist character, help motivate clients towards the goal of reduction in suicidal thoughts. These approaches are also easier to teach compared to many other therapies.

From a clinical perspective, it may not be right for all clients, but as a first line of defence against suicide, it is worth a project training staff in this approach so the client can experience a coordinated response to their situation. When all staff are re-enforcing the client's recovery in the same way, it strengthens and accelerates behavioural change.

Breaking the Social Isolation Factor

Brodsky, Spruch-Feiner, and Stanley (2018) reviewed how suicide prevention research informs implementation of clinical care when those most at risk present. They summarised the area of delivery to include risk assessment, means restriction, evidence-based treatments, population screening combined with chain of care, monitoring, and follow-up.

They discussed how the USA National Action Alliance for Suicide Prevention presents the Zero Suicide (ZS) model to coordinate a multilevel approach implementing evidence-based practices. A review of 1800 studies clearly suggested the paramount importance of evidence-based clinical practice.

There were, however, huge holes in the proposals. The USA can be a brutal country with poor regard for social support of the average working-class person and especially the poor. It can have a poor level of social medicine supply as it is largely a private health fund driven system. It has some of the highest levels of poverty, addiction, homelessness, murder and crime due to its social and political systems. The concept of psychosocial approaches virtually ignores the clients' reintegration and resocialisation back into society.

Again, we come back to the fact that SGD minority stress and high suicide ideation are mainly driven by social, workplace, familial, medical, and legal rejection and shunning of people from those groups. Isolated clinical interventions without re-socialisation will never produce a zero-suicide rate. Involving family and friends simply to monitor the client and clinical follow-up alone is not social reintegration. Many people from SGD groups do not have those networks.

Social reintegration is teaching the client resilience and motivating them to re-engage with others. Humans are pack animals and do best when they have the social support of the groups they create and are part of on a daily basis. Increased isolation creates poor mental health in people from SGD groups, particularly when that is driven by social, institutional and governmental sexism and genderism. Increased positive socialisation creates community, social support, validation of self, others and the value of life-reducing suicidal ideation.

Isolation, loneliness, rejection and feelings of being excluded from one's peers can be key in the deterioration of mental health. That isolation can happen in many forms: simply locking oneself away and not seeing others, living in remote places, having no friends, being ex-communicated from family, friends or colleagues, being positioned as the outsider in social groups and being a member of misunderstood groups like SGD groups.

Intelligence, education or pre-existing social dominance give no advantage to the individual when they become isolated or are confined in small groups. It should not be presumed that previous life advantages preclude suicidal ideation when someone is exposed to SGD minority stress.

The use of social programs and outreach workers to help reintegrate SGD people back into groups that will accept and welcome them can be very useful in suicide recovery. It is well worth projects setting aside funds for client socialisation facilitation. This also introduces clients to the concept that they are not alone and can be accepted for exactly who and what they are, giving them space away from situations or people that may be exacerbating the minority stress. Remedial therapeutic approaches alone do not solve the problem of isolation and social ostracisation, but social connections and attachments generally do lower depression and thereby the risk of suicide.

It is worth considering a duality here in that clients can be guided by social workers to special support networks around their sex and gender status, and to community programs and social groups for people seeking to meet others. Most governments already have cost-benefit analyses, return on investment research and statistics around social programs that can be paralleled across for the provision of needs in depressed and suicidal SGD groups.

References

ACON For Health, Australia. (2020). https://www.acon.org.au/who-we-are-here-for/tgd-people/

Ashley, A. (2016). *First lady.* Blake Publishing

Australasian College of Emergency Medicine (2019). "A state of crisis": Data shows blow outs for mental health care. Retrieved from https://acem.org.au/News/Oct-2018/A-state-of-crisis%E2%80%9D-Data-shows-blow-outs-for-ment

Bach, N. (2018, October 22). What the Trump Administration's proposed gender rules changes could mean for trans people. *Fortune.* Retrieved from http://fortune.com/2018/10/22/transgender-rights-trump-administration/

Blackstone Chambers. (2018, June 22). R (Christie Elan-Cane) v Secretary of State for the Home Department. Retrieved from www.blackstonechambers.com/news/r-christie-elan-cane-v-secretary-state-home-department/

Brodsky, B., Spruch-Feiner, A., & Stanley, B. (2018). The zero suicide model: Applying evidence-based suicide prevention practices to clinical care. *Frontiers in Psychiatry.* Retrieved from https://doi.org/10.3389/fpsyt.2018.00033

Bryan, C. & Rudd, M. (2018). *Brief cognitive-behavioral therapy for suicide prevention* (1st ed). The Guilford Press

Campbell, L.C. (1997). *Lady Colin Campbell: Autobiography.* Little, Brown & Company.

Colapinto, J. (2000). *As nature made him: The boy who was raised as a girl.* HarperCollins Publishers

Cross, D. (2018, October 28). Perth hospitals declare emergency mental health code yellow after 'ugly week.' *The Sydney Morning Herald.* Retrieved from https://www.smh.com.au/lifestyle/health-and-wellness/perth-hospitals-declare-emergency-mental-health-code-yellow-after-ugly-week-20181026-p50c9p.html

Department of Health, Victoria. (2014). Transgender and gender diverse health and wellbeing. Retrieved from https://www2.health.vic.gov.au/about/publications/researchandreports/Transgender-and-gender-diverse-health-and-wellbeing

Haydar, N. (2017, April 16). Safe Schools program ditched in NSW, to be replaced by wider anti-bullying. *ABC News.* Retrieved from https://www.abc.net.au/news/2017-04-16/safe-schools-program-ditched-in-nsw/8446680

High Court of Australia. (2014). Registrar of Births, Deaths and Marriages v. Norrie, HCA 11.

Lahood, G. [Deme Perez] (2012). Intersexion Documentary. Retrieved from https://www.youtube.com/watch?v=QQdOp3COfSs

Los Angeles LGBT Centre. (2020). https://lalgbtcenter.org/

about-the-center

McCloskey, D. (1999). *Crossing: A memoir* (1st ed). University of Chicago Press.

Money, J. (1996, January 1). *Man & woman, boy & girl: Gender identity from conception to maturity* (The Master Work Series). Jason Aronson, Inc.

Potaka, E. (2018, March 27). Fake doctors, banned drugs, risky procedures: Inside Australia's backyard beauty clinics. *SBS*. Retrieved from www.sbs.com.au/news/the-feed/fake-doctors-banned-drugs-risky-procedures-inside-australia-s-backyard-beauty-clinics

QMUNITY, Canada, sourced February, 2019. https://qmunity.ca/get-support/couselling/

Ramsay, M. (2017, October 1). Colombians in search of beauty risk death from 'cowboy' surgery. *The Guardian*. Retrieved from https://www.theguardian.com/world/2017/sep/30/colombians-in-hunt-for-beauty-risk-death-cowboy-surgery

Salam, R., Haroon, S., Ahmed, H., Das, J. & Bhutta, Z. (2014). Impact of community-based interventions on HIV knowledge, attitudes, and transmission. *Infectious Diseases of Poverty*. Retrieved from https://www.ncbi.nlm.nih.gov/pmc/articles/PMC4132935/

The Center New York, USA. (2020). https://gaycenter.org/recovery-health/health/hiv-aids/

Chapter 10:
Screening for Suicidation

One of the obvious and well-recognised risks for suicide is a history of suicidal thoughts and attempted suicides (Park et al., 2018). Acute stress reactions are particularly brought on by the presence of SGD minority stress, and health professionals need to be constantly vigilant of those suicide risk factors. The threat of that stress does not disappear because someone has not completed suicide or because they may appear to have become comfortable in who and what they are.

Fawcett (2012) states the likelihood of suicide increases further with the presence of co-morbidities such as schizophrenia, borderline personality disorder, bipolar disorders, eating disorders, addiction, acute stress disorders and particularly mood disorders. In these cases of high suicide risk and complex co-morbidities, plus SGD minority stress, institutionalised assessment with clients in extreme crisis may be an option. Being placed on a nursing suicide watch may be the cautious option even though it may result in the risk of losing rapport with the client. Fawcett refers to these groups being categorised as acute high risk and sometimes chronic high risk.

The situation with complex comorbidities and high suicide risk also gives rise to the issues of duty of care of harm to self or others and professional obligations to clients and the public to protect life. As professionals, at times, we need to take action to comply with the laws of the land to protect ourselves. After each successful suicide, an inquest may require us to account for our professionalism and the client's best interests, and we must also act according to our professional codes by which we agree to practise.

For clients without acute or chronic mental pathologies, but who have simply moved to suicidality due to SGD minority stress or an existential crisis around their sex and/or gender status, we need to start asking a range of questions of the situation and client. Here establishing rapport and maintaining it is paramount so the client will feel safe and open up. We must, however, be mindful to remain objective in order to assess them, without personal involvement bias in screening for suicidal thoughts, motivation, behaviour, emotional dysregulation and in formulating a treatment plan. Good and effective health professional practices are always constant detective work.

Screening with Tests
Using tests and assessment tools can give false positives or false negatives at the best of times when dealing with the average populations (Gregory, 2013). Results can be rendered null and void due to all sorts of user and administration errors. We also have to consider that many clients confabulate and at times respond with outright lies in order to fulfil a hidden agenda or sometimes because of passive-aggressive anger towards the tester. For tests to work well, the recipient needs to demonstrate disclosure, compliance and voluntariness, not coercive co-operation. There must also be reasonable cognitive comprehension, but when people have moved into suicidal ideation, they do not fit that criterion so errors are inevitable.

Misdiagnosis of mental disorders in people from SGD groups is not only common but probably standard for a large majority of cases. When you apply standardised tests and assessment tools, possibly designed by white middle-class American males, to a culturally disadvantaged group experiencing minority stress, extraneous variables will arise.

These include a history of abuse, social isolation, harassment, economic disadvantage, workplace exclusion, familial hostility, linguistic and cultural differences, legal and religious persecution, intergenerational medical abuse, and sex and gender minority stress. No design can compensate for all of those factors. Pretending those tests can measure accurately is not in the best interests of the client as cultural and subcultural distortion is present, particularly if test coerciveness is present or the patient complies to get other people to leave them alone. So true rapport and co-operation is highly unlikely to exist.

Different cultures attach different values to clinical testing but mainly they are also used for the benefit of the clinician to help them be legally safe, just as much as a record of the client's experience. They are also used for funding and treatment justification and at times a misdiagnosis may be given simply to gain funding for a client's other needs. When a client gains a diagnosis, they can then move into a state of acting out the diagnosis short- and long-term, even when the misdiagnosis is influenced by cultural misunderstanding.

Make no mistake, people from SGD groups can have their own cultures and sub-cultures with history, affiliations, stories, solutions, hostilities and psychological gestalts. These experiences are intrapersonal and shared interpersonally as well as on the internet, which may be outside the health professional's experience.

We must also consider that test results are transient, a photograph in time of a person's state of mind at that moment, and should not necessarily be a predictor for long-term treatment plans. Spikes that show in results during short-term trauma can be subject to stereotyping threats and can be absent a week later when circumstances change. Results disclosed to someone who is suicidal can be misinterpreted by the client with unintended meaning, creating a self-fulfilling prophecy that there really is something very wrong with them. Results from official mental health tests can, at times, be seen as reasons for suicide by the client.

Let us look again at the administration of the MMPI given to trans people. The MMPI-2 was administered to 108 French transsexuals applying for standardised sex reassignment procedures in a public university hospital between 2007–2010 (Bonierbale et al., 2016). The main finding of the study was that the sample group were relatively free of pathology. The errors and distortions that happened here, however, are that many French transsexuals lie to doctors.

I lived and worked in France, including with SGD groups in Paris, so know the routine of telling other people's stories that clients followed to get clinicians to prescribe hormones and gain access to surgery. Since I worked in the community, I was privy to the stories that many clients faked to gain access to clinical care. Many of the clinics used a psychoanalytical approach, so they were basically looking for a pass or fail story from the patients to permit or deny transition. France's overly patriarchal attitude to transition meant patients learnt the script that they believed the doctors wanted to hear to access medical help. The script was repeated like a parrot until clinics gave the clients what they wanted.

Since no acute stress due to minority stress showed up in the MMPI-2 test results, we can see testing was often a pantomime. Trans people in France have suffered profound, traumatic minority stress, which should have conclusively showed up in the results.

Diametrically-opposed results were obtained by Hepp et al. (2005) who found a high level of psychiatric comorbidity in people identified as experiencing gender dysphoria. Other studies have given equally as wide a range of results. So, what we are really seeing is test design, administration and interpretation errors, which make such tests unreliable in SGD populations, except in the presence of extreme acute psycho-pathology, which would be registered by default, due to its extreme and blatantly obvious behavioural nature.

There is also the matter of confidentiality and electronic records. Countries are trying to move to electronic medical records that remain with a person for life. Misinterpretation of mental illness through the mis-administration of tests like MMPI-2 and depression scales can have detrimental effects on the client's future prospects for education and employment, so it is unsurprising that many test-takers lie.

Suicide Gene

Despite the quest of some geneticists to find a suicide gene, it would be impossible to find one because people complete suicide for so many different reasons and in different circumstances. While certain genetic variances may create psychological disturbances and instability that can give rise to physical and mental dysregulation and even mental illness, suicide is generally an "existential crisis of being" or a perceived solution to what the person considers is an intolerable situation.

Prewarning Signs

There may be prewarning signs that lead up to suicidal behaviours such as depression, anxiety, panic attacks, post-traumatic stress disorder, appearing withdrawn, a decline in self-care, disengagement from social contact, self-imposed isolation, loss of interest in activities, failure to engage in conversation, feelings of hopelessness and helplessness, out-of-character impulsive behaviours and anger, inability to future pace during conversation, negative self talk, sense of worthlessness, recent experiences of being bullied or being subject to violence, insomnia, loss of relationship or friends, failure to keep appointments, the giving away of possessions, substance abuse, emotional trauma, major affective disorders and chronic mental illness.

People from SGD groups often cannot and do not disclose information around their sex or gender experience for fear of friends, families and healthcare professionals' reactions. They may fear psychiatric admission, being forced onto medications they do not want or being rejected and stigmatised.

Because they have run out of stamina to deal with the overwhelming escalating suicide ideation and negative emotions, they may just be giving up on life. Along with that, they may be experiencing shame and guilt about being suicidal, which adds another layer of difficulty on top of simply being from a SGD group.

Families, friends, carers and health professionals can miss these prewarning suicide risk factors. Since indicators can be multiple and in any combinations, it can be hard for others to keep track when the client is keeping information secret. So many people attempt suicide without outward prewarning signs and those close to them are left wondering what they missed.

Suicide Plan

One of the lines of questioning in suicide screening to detect the levels of suicidal ideation is to ask if the person has ever had a suicide plan. If they have never thought suicide through to the extent of a plan, it is likely any suicidal ideations are emotively driven by a present perceived situation, events or trauma. It may be necessary to probe further to find the source of that distress as diplomatically as possible.

Sometimes the stress reaction of any suicide threat or attempt is part of an affective mood disorder, particularly Borderline Personality Disorder (BPD). This can only be verified by outside sources of information as this disorder may not be evident at a first meeting. It is easy for professionals to initially miss the signs of personality disorders and mental illness.

When someone has had a suicide plan, ruminated on it

for a while, had more than one plan, had previous attempts or long-time thoughts of suicide, it is a clear sign of long-term depression. In these cases, a client may try to hide some of that history from you, perceiving your questions as interference and a threat to them maintaining their suicide plan. Such clients often keep diaries recording their inner turmoil and dark thoughts. You may ask if they have anything in their diaries or thoughts that they might like to share to enable you to help them.

As paradoxical as it may seem, sometimes having a suicide plan may be a way for the client to put off suicide until a later time, but when you question the client, they may feel challenged and proceed to execute the plan. The more detailed and obsessed they are with the plan, the higher the risk that they may actually execute it at some stage.

One of the ways to ask defensive clients questions is to use what I call the "idiot questioner approach". You profess ignorance and being out of your depth with the situation and ask their help to understand and react responsibly. In other words, you turn the tables to them helping you, not you helping them. When someone knows great distress, they are more likely to have empathy with others in distress and may be willing to help you. For instance, the man about to jump off the bridge may stop to save the child walking out in front of the traffic. By breaking the mental suicide state, it can change the suicidal person into the rescuer role of saviour and empower them.

Screening Tests
Despite what I have said about test fallibility, you may legally or contractually be obliged to use them. Different disciplines tend to use different suicide screening instruments from psychiatry to nursing, social work, psychology, psychotherapy and counselling, according to what signs and symptoms are being observed. Each of us is looking for different indications

of suicidal thoughts and their severity. Such tests are used not only to screen but also to fit in with time frames and clinical management.

The circumstances of administering such tests are rarely ideal and often we are unable to glean large amounts of qualitative information in order to build rapport with the clients. A practitioner may also be obliged to use such tests due to instructions from a line manager or to comply with departmental, institutional or clinical regulations.

Wherever possible, a practitioner will always gather higher-quality information from structured active interviews where rapport is built, lowering the client's defence mechanisms, so they disclose more information than simply administering a pen and pencil or computer test. This allows observation of body language, voice tone, respiratory dysregulation, skin colour changes, defensive reactions, distraction, dissociation, passive-aggressive statements and behaviour, eye pattern detection of confabulation, memory and informational management coding, and indications of voluntariness and co-operation. The practitioner is also able to extend the threads of answers in order to gather a deeper understanding of the client's psychological and emotional state.

What You Need to Consider

An individual may experience chronic long-term, low-grade suicidal thoughts throughout their life, suffering a persistent sense of depression, disappointment, hopelessness or fear of life. These people are aware of those persistent, underlying suicidal thoughts and they may never have talked about them and rarely reveal them to others. In classic psychoanalytical terms, Freud (1922/2009) referred to this as the Thanatos instinct, the death drive. Those suicidal thoughts can become attached to sex and/or gender issues or the person can experience multiple triggers due to complex trauma or a general pessimistic attitude to life and their grim projected imagined future.

Others may experience the acute onset of suicidal thoughts due to simple trauma and loss: the loss of a body part, loved one, dignity, financial position, public or socially integrity. Those thoughts are suddenly overwhelming for the person and they are often confused and panicked about what is happening to them.

With the right questioning, you can observe how distressed and disorientated the client has become, which may even be quite out of character for them. Suddenly their issues around sex and/or gender become psychologically and emotionally enlarged in their mind, causing them to become overwhelmed, afraid and move towards suicidality.

People who experience post-traumatic stress disorder (PTSD) may have a sudden onset of suicidal thoughts when they are triggered into the regressive panic state where they are replaying the past or multiple past traumas in their mind. They also experience an uncontrollable emotional defence response that can render them quite incapable of carrying out ordinary everyday tasks; they freeze. Many people who experience sex and/or gender diversity report having experienced physical, mental and sexual abuse. In enquiring about this past trauma, the practitioner must be careful not to trigger or overwhelm clients with their memories of past trauma, which could compound thoughts of suicide.

A kind of suicidal state you will encounter as a health professional is the aberration. It is when someone commits suicide quite unexpectedly with no warning whatsoever. Clinicians, carers, relatives and friends will say they never saw it coming because the person showed no signs of what was about to happen. In these cases, it may be possible to trace back triggers but, in some cases, we may never know why the person ended their life. This is common in the general population and in SGD groups.

The cry-for-help suicide attempt is the person reaching out

for attention. They may not feel their issues are being heard or being taken seriously enough by others. They may even not have the words or language to describe their experiences, how they feel or what is happening to them. Young people, in particular, may have no experience or vocabulary that describes their perceived or actual sex and gender difference. The only way they can see to be noticed is to scream out for help by going to the brink of actual suicide, then draw back in fear in front of others, so their pains and frustrations are noticed.

Accidental suicide is common when a person needs to act out suicide as a cry for help, but unfortunately, they do not execute their rescue plan well or misjudge when and how to draw back from suicide. Since they successfully suicide, we can only surmise they did not intend to actually suicide all the way to death. In this case, they do not leave a suicide note because they intended to talk about it with others once they were rescued. They may even have never mentioned their sex or gender issues and those are only later discovered by the material they leave behind.

Suicidal people with mental health problems such as active schizophrenia, bipolar disorder and BPD may constantly threaten and attempt suicide. This behaviour can be equally as prevalent when they are institutionalised as when they are living in the community. They can demand high clinical attention and some institutions may not take them as they are too disturbing on the wards. This client should always have a multi-disciplinary and focused care plan and it is unwise for singular practitioners to attempt to handle these cases alone. Often, the client's sex or gender issues have not been taken seriously and it can be hard for health professionals to sort out which are the prevalent drivers of suicide.

Iatrogenic drug-induced suicide is common. Anti-depressants, anti-psychotics, sedative depressants and prescribed stimulants should all carry warnings of suicidal thoughts and behaviours for some users. The side-effects can not only be suicidal thoughts but also complete derangement and psychotic episodes. Patients, parents or carers are rarely made fully aware of these potential side-effects because the prescriber is under pressure from their associations to prescribe those drugs and can even be found guilty of negligence for not prescribing them. The iatrogenic-induced psychotic decompression can unleash a flood of emotions around any sex or gender issues that the person finds frightening and overwhelming and this can cause them to move to suicide.

Self-harming thoughts and behaviours are common in SGD groups when people are disconnected from their bodies or have considerable difficulties acting out sex or gender preference. There can be an undying sense of shame and self-hatred arising from a sense of worthlessness, often initiated by social rejection or being told to keep what they are secret and not public. Accumulated shame and guilt from religious or social programming over a person's sex or gender status can lead to self-harming, which can accelerate and amplify suicidal thoughts.

Self-harming such as cutting is also frequently used as a control mechanism by clients. Like eating disorders it may be perceived as something they can control when other parts of their lives seem uncontrollable.

People bullied about their sex or gender often do not tell their immediate carers, family or friends. They may be afraid to disclose and if they put words to the experience, the trauma runs the risk of becoming more real for them. So, some people keep their experience to themselves until they are unable to cope anymore and they move towards suicide as a relief from their present circumstances. The emotional overwhelm they experience blocks their cognitive problem-solving skills.

Some people confused about their sex or gender who have suddenly found out they are intersex or have problems dealing with the reality of their sex or gender situation may suicide. In general, clinicians only see a person for a short time, deliver information and then the client leaves with what can be shocking news that overwhelms them. They may be angry with themselves and others, and the shock and anger may precipitate suicidal thoughts for fear they will not be able to cope with their reality.

As noted earlier in this book, many people from SGD groups suffer profound clinical, social, institutional, familial, religious and educational and workplace abuse. It is often not just abuse in one area of their lives but multi-locational and multi-faceted. There is frequently no refuge to retreat to so there is no respite from the constant onslaught of abuse that can lead to deep depression and suicidal thoughts. People who carry out this abuse believe it is their right under free speech and fail to understand the complex trauma experience it sets up in people with sex or gender issues. This rolling stone collection of traumas eventually gathers such a large load of complex traumas that the person can often see suicide as the only door to peace.

There are those from SGD groups who are economically disadvantaged. The pressures of paying for life-long medical expenses or the economic toll when they have been excluded from society can be overwhelming. This can lead people to access non-qualified medical help or black market medications and to undergoing unsanctioned cosmetic procedures. The consequence of these procedures can lead to life-threatening medical situations, disfigurement and, at times, people trying to carry out surgery on themselves and their friends. The pain, ill-health and possibility of death that follows can lead some to suicide.

When as a health professional you screen for reasons behind the person's suicidal ideation, you need to screen for all of the above without traumatising or re-traumatising the client, while practising a high degree of active listening, allowing the person space for catharsis and to tell their story.

Asking the Suicide Question

For healthcare workers who work with people from SGD groups, it is important to remember how vulnerable these populations can be in the wider world as a minority. For the short time we see them, we are only ever able to gather a reasonably small amount of information on their orientation in the world, so it is possible to miss many influences that they may encounter.

Suicidal thoughts lie at different levels of the consciousness depending on how prevalent they may be at a particular time of a person's life. They may be triggered by another person, group, event, incident or emotions to elevate them higher in conscious awareness, increasing present suicide risk. As Jung (1970) proposed, each part of our personalities comes and goes from consciousness according to our criteria of needs in the moment. While we as clinicians want to talk to the subpersonality that wants to kill the client, we do not want it to be overly dominant, intrusive or causing coping strategy dysregulation and psychotic decompression.

So, in the quest to gather information, we also elicit other sub-personalities in order to counteract the death wish and desensitise the client to the shadow part of themselves. Amelioration always begins during observation not after.

It is essential to ask the client if they have experienced any suicidal thoughts and when. This must be phrased with a high degree of tact and diplomacy in order not to render the client's defence mechanisms active, trigger or lead them to believe that you may think them mentally unstable just because they are from a SGD group.

You might say:

"I hope you don't mind me asking. And I'm just checking in with you. You see, asking questions like this is part of my job in caring for you, and I do have to ask these questions

of many people, and I have to ask them anyway. Have
you ever had or do you have any suicidal thoughts at the
moment? And of course, I will check in with you from time
to time about this and you know you can always talk to me if
you need to and ask for help, don't you?"

These are what are called open questions with validators, invitations and qualifiers. The question is open because it requires an interpretation from the client. You are validating the need to ask the question, inviting an answer and qualifying the person as being important enough to be asked such a caring question.

If the person has expressed they have had suicidal thoughts, you always need to ask if they have a plan about how they might complete suicide. I know this sounds like it might be an enquiry too far, but it will tell you how progressed the suicidal thoughts might be and if they have already taken any action towards suicide. You cannot skip this question.

Most suicide is driven by a spur-of-the-moment emotional overload, but other people who attempt suicide may have been planning the action over a long time and waiting until what they think is the right time. Thinking and fantasising about suicide is not the same as having taken action to make that happen, which indicates more serious intentions.

What you are also doing is extending the questioning and giving the client permission and a space to talk about what they have or are experiencing, which is not available to them in ordinary society. This allows them to have a sense of significance and being heard, and the knowledge that someone is taking notice of their distress. It is proactive listening.

Having opened up the discussion, you can ask the client to rate their level of desire to complete suicide using a subjective unit of disturbance (SUD) scale of 0–10, with 0 being "do not want to complete suicide at all" and 10 being "feeling like completing suicide at this moment".

You could say:

*"How much do you want to complete suicide at the moment?
On a scale of 0 to 10, with 10 being high and 0 being low,
how much do you want to complete suicide at the moment?"*

This will help tell you how much you need to pay attention to the suicide issue with this client. Since the average person does not want to commit suicide at all, you should treat anything above a 5 as a suicide emergency, and not just lingering fantasies of suicide that need attention to discuss their existential nature.

Other important questions are about frequency. While these are open questions and are directly screening for triggers, you are also allowing the client to identify their time triggers.

You might say:

*"How often do those thoughts occur?'
"Are they at any particular times?"*

You are involved in two processes here. The first is the screening for how serious suicidality is at the moment or an identifiable time of risk. The second is that you are asking the client to challenge themselves about how serious they are about suicide by looking at how carefully they have thought about the suicide process.

These are difficult questions for us to ask as health professionals because they tap into our own existential doubts about how effective we can be working with the client. Part of working in healthcare is that we know we can help so many people but there are always the ones we cannot help, which gives us self-doubt, particularly if we are new to working in the area of sex and gender diversity. However, we must ask these questions in a calm, self-assured and empathic way.

You may not have had suicide screening training, nor have the confidence or you may not think this is part of your job description. You may be influenced by your own religious beliefs. You may even be daunted by the politics around asking such questions of people from SGD groups. However, as carers, we do have a duty to monitor and observe whether those thoughts or actions are manifesting in clients, without judgement.

Such questions should always be asked when you are facing someone, still, in a quiet voice, sitting down opposite the person, with eye contact so you can see the physical response and whether the client recoils at the question in a defensive response. If answers indicate risk, you need to gently enquire a little more with a more open question to get to the root of their response.

It is equally as important to ask the questions around suicidal thoughts with these clients regularly. They may at times not be doing well with their issues around their sex or gender because of their co-morbidities. All health carers involved need to be observant for potential suicidal behaviour, language and patterns, alerting other professionals if they think the client is at risk.

What is notable here is that all people from SGD groups who exhibit suicidation should be assessed for PTSD and Trauma I, II and III. As you can see from the reporting in this book, not to find trauma in those populations would likely be an assessment error. I have never in my own career encountered a suicidal patient from this group of clients who has not experienced trauma in one form or another. To try and treat suicidal thoughts without addressing and remediating that trauma will not render results or only short-term results. This might not be possible in an emergency situation but it will need to be addressed in the treatment plan.

More Investigative Questions

If the client is already known to you, some questions may be superfluous, but it is important to get a present-tense perspective if there are indications of suicide risk. Some questions can be open and some binary (yes or no). Some clients may be angry about talking to you and will often answer in single answers, so try and increase the number of open questions, allowing them to talk. It does not matter if they stray off-topic sometimes or rant, as they are talking and opening up, but just gently bring them back to the conversation.

Begin with:

> *"I wonder if you might be so kind as to help me understand what you are experiencing. I would like to ask you for some more information so I can help."*

Present Emotional State
→ Tell me how have you felt lately?
→ Do you know why you feel that way?
→ Have you felt that way for long and if so, how long?
→ Have you ever felt like that before?

Environment Pressure From Others
→ How are things at work or school?
→ Is anyone putting any pressure on you or treating you unkindly?
→ Is anyone bullying you or making rude comments about you?
→ Why do you think they might be behaving that way?

Home Situation
→ How are things at home?
→ Are you happy when you are around your family?
→ Do you feel they support you and do you feel safe?

→ Is there anyone in the family you have problems with and why?

Looking for Sex Dysphoria
→ How do you feel about your body?
→ How do you feel about what sex you are?
→ What do you like and what do you dislike about your body?
→ Is there anything you would like to change?

Looking for Gender Dysphoria
→ Are you happy acting as male/female or other (whichever is appropriate)?
→ Are you happy with the way other people see your gender performance?
→ Are there changes you might have been thinking about with your gender performance?
→ How would you like others to see you?

Impulsivity
→ Do you think you are someone who thinks about things carefully?
→ Do you act and then think about it or think about something carefully before you act?
→ Would you say you are a patient person?
→ Are there any times when you do something suddenly and then find yourself in trouble?

Frustration
→ Are you angry with anyone at the moment?
→ Why are you angry with them and for how long will you be angry with them?
→ Are you angry with yourself?
→ Why are you angry with yourself and how long has this been like this?

Trauma

→ Is there anything that has really upset you lately?
→ Did anything happen that was difficult to deal with that distressed you?
→ Has anyone hurt you recently or in the past?
→ Are you afraid of any situation?

Self-Harm

→ Have there been any times when you have thought about hurting yourself?
→ Are there any times when you have hurt yourself?
→ How often and for how long has that occurred?
→ Have you ever told anyone about that before?

Suicide Attempts

→ Are there any times you have thoughts about ending your life?
→ Are there any times when you have tried to end your life?
→ What do you think made you think and act that way?
→ Who have you told about that before and what was their reaction?

Resource Mining

→ Did you know everyone gets really upset and feels down sometimes?
→ Are you aware that sometimes many people feel like they don't want to live anymore?
→ Did you know that people can get past that, become stronger and find ways to have a happy life, people just like you?
→ What do you do to solve problems?

Looking for Support

→ Can you name four friends for me?
→ What do you like about each of them?

→ How often do you see them and how do they support you or you support them?

→ How do you have fun with them?

Offering Help

→ What would you like help with?

→ What help you do need right now?

→ How do you think we might be able to help you with that?

→ If we helped you, would you be prepared to work to be part of the solution?

It is important when screening someone that you come with soft questions first to build rapport and then ask the more difficult questions so that the client feels safe in answering those without judgement. Always end the questions on a positive note, giving the client a sense they are important and worthy. Never finish screening with an open wound showing. Do not over-promise but leave the client with a sense of possibilities and hope – that if you cannot help them, you can refer them to someone who might be able to.

The Suicide Note

Much or little is disclosed in a suicide note. It is the tool of someone who actually intends to complete suicide and a testament to their final thoughts. It is not a record of their life or relationships but a record of their final emotional catharsis. It may be full of anger, blame, resentment, apology, regret or sentiments of love, appreciation and thanks for their life. It may even give instructions to those who find it or the people they leave alive.

Not everyone who completes suicide leaves a suicide note, only those who really consider their actions and plan before they carry out their suicide. The note may even serve as a final reminder that they lived and a last connection with the life they leave behind.

The note may be a comforter for those left behind (lovers, friends, relatives, therapists) or a poetic justification of the act, but it will not always give the reasons the person took their life. Many people left behind preserve the note as a memento of the last moments the person was alive and it becomes their last connection to them. But not too much should be read into the note because there may be many stressors that lead a person towards suicide and far too many to state or remember in a note. There may not even be any mention of their sex and gender issues in the note. It is important to remember that it may even have been other issues too that pushed them over the edge to suicide.

Report Writing

Time is the enemy of all practitioners as we have so many facets to our jobs that we have to complete. We are always time-poor and under caseload pressure. In writing screening reports and making referrals, remember to write the report as if it was going to be read by the client's grandmother, because under freedom of information access, it may well be at some stage. Over-interpretation is the curse of screening.

The whole point of a screening process is to determine what is in the best interest of the client, not how clever the clinician is, even though you may be good at what you practise. Clearly state what you found and what help the client may need. Do not overly pathologise people from SGD groups as they are already under attack from large sectors of society.

Call upon the help of more than one agency if necessary and stretch the permissibility to refer people to charities and self-help advocacy groups if you think the person could benefit. Many people from SGD groups struggle with poverty and cannot afford private care, but they can gain enormously from the voluntary sector.

Gatekeeper Suicide Screening

Gatekeeper suicide screening has become a popular system for spotting people who may be at risk of suicide in communities (Burnette et al., 2015). It is being used by the military, ethnic communities and communities that have an organised hierarchy and structures. Individuals in key positions, including at least one health professional, are trained in the gatekeeper system to refer people who show signs of possible suicide risk to mental health professionals.

Despite enthusiasm from small communities, this system is not suitable for SGD groups unless those persons are in the military, institutional systems or communities. Many people from SGD groups are stealth, not out publicly about their sex or gender status, so they can be unreachable and unobservable.

Children

In working with suicidal children, home assessments are a necessary part of the comprehensive assessment of suicide risk. This must always include a social worker who can assess family dynamics and assess whether the family is supportive of the child or part of the problems that led to the child's depression and increased suicide risk. If the family's behavioural dynamics do increase the risk of suicide, an assessment of whether the child should be temporarily removed from the home should be carried out. If the risk is found to be due to family dynamics, the child should be removed at least temporarily.

When a home environment is toxic to a child who is suicidal, there is due cause for removal and supportive foster care placement until family psychodynamics can be changed. Sometimes the removal of a vulnerable child can be devastating to the child even when they know the family is the problem that is driving them to suicide. The reality of keeping a child in the family home of origin, though, is not the best choice when that environment is a threat to their well-being. A gentler option is sometimes to place the child with supportive relatives.

It is also important to consider that it may be difficult to observe a child in a toxic home environment where the child is repressed. In such an emergency, like potential suicide, it may be much easier to assess the child when they are, albeit temporarily, removed from a toxic environment to give clearer indications of the problems.

There is much controversy around removal of children at risk from families of origin, particularly when the family may have certain beliefs and claim religious freedom to raise their child as they see fit. However, minors deserve the protection of the state, and it is the duty of care of health professionals to preserve life and recognise that children from SGD groups may experience bullying within their own families.

Training Parents to Screen Children from SGD Groups for Suicidation

We can consider the Telethon Kids Institute in Australia published a study called The Mental Health Experiences and Care Pathways of Trans Young People (Strauss et al., 2017). The information was gathered from trans-identified children and their parents, with 859 participants. The children's thoughts and behaviours were reported. Of the participants, 91.3% had previously wanted to self-harm, 66.7% within the last 12 months; 79.7% had self-harmed, 43.6% within the last year; 62.8% had had reckless behaviour, 33% within the past year; 82.4% had had thoughts of suicide, 48.8% within the past year; 48.1% had attempted suicide, 16.1% within the past year. We need to take note of this reporting.

Parents, caregivers and families of children from SGD groups fit into a number of categories: those who fully embrace the situation, those who resist the situation, those who hide the situation as a secret and do not want it known publicly, and those who are incompetent and abusive towards the child.

Health professionals treating children from SGD groups also need to make help available to the family and make them aware of the risk of self-harming and suicide in those children. As part of treatment of the child, it needs to be strongly emphasised that the parents also need to attend family sessions where they are taught how to spot the risk of suicide in their children and support them.

Considering the level of risk of self-harm to children from SGD groups, if the parents refuse, thereby ignoring that risk of suicide, then the child should be placed on an at-risk children's social services register. The well-being and protection of the child should always supersede any beliefs, religious or otherwise, of the parent or family.

Teach parents and carers to ask something like:

> *"Hey, I just wanted to check in with you. How are things going today? Is there anything you need or want to talk about because we can talk about anything you want? You know that, don't you? We are here to care for you and love you and see you are happy. Have you had any suicidal thoughts? Is there anything you need or want to talk about?"*

For children, it is important for carers and parents to talk to their wards regularly so that those disturbing thoughts do not become the unspoken secrets that are missed. It is wise to advise parents to adopt this strategy to monitor their minor's mental state, through proactively parenting.

Here teachers and extended carers need to be careful that they are acting on the instruction of healthcare professionals and not simply taking it upon themselves to fulfil those roles.

When children become suicidal, it is important to refer

them to child specialists or practitioners experienced in working children who understand SGD groups. It is wise to be discerning about the professionals they are exposed to as there are many practitioners who will pathologise the child's experience of being sex and/or gender diverse.

For example, an American group of paediatricians created a small group called the American College of Paediatricians (ACP). In 2010, the ACP sent out 1400 letters to school district superintendents promoting reparative therapy that tries to convert children to behave in a stereotypical heteronormative fashion, which has been shown to be harmful and dangerous by heightening the risk of suicide (Turban, 2017).

Parents also have to be careful about what public information children from SGD groups are exposed to. In the UK, Baroness Nicholson of the House of Lords released a letter that she sent to the chairman of the large chain of shops Marks & Spencer (House of Lords Member Baroness Nicholson, 2020), She tried to persuade the board that allowing trans people and children to use the female changing rooms was dangerous and exposed women to violence. Her letter was made public and put fear into SGD groups of children who used the store, as well as parents of children from non-SGD groups.

The constant public bombardment of attacks on the rights of SGD groups by right-wing, uneducated public figures on television and in the media can lead to high levels of anxiety and fear in children from SGD groups. It is important for parents and carers to filter such information that children are exposed to in order for them to feel safe and valued.

What is dropped into the mind of the child will remain there for life so be sure they get the message loud and clear that they are worth listening to and caring for, regardless of their sex or gender presentation.

References

Bonierbale, M., Baumstarck, K., Maquigneau, A., Gorin-Lazard, A., Boyer, L., Loundou, A., Auquier, P. & Lancon, C. (2016). MMPI-2 Profile of French transsexuals: The role of sociodemographic and clinical factors. A cross-sectional design. *Scientific Reports.* doi: 10.1038/srep24281

Burnette, C., Ramchand, R. & Ayer, L. (2015). Gatekeeper training for suicide prevention. A theoretical model and review of the empirical literature. *Rand Health Quarterly.* Retrieved from https://www.ncbi.nlm.nih.gov/pmc/articles/PMC5158249/

Fawcett, J. (2012). *The neurobiological basis of suicide.* CRC Press/Taylor & Francis.

Freud, S. (2009). *Beyond the pleasure principle* (1st ed.). Dover Publications. (Original work published 1922)

Gregory, R. (2013). Psychological testing: History, principles, and applications. *Pearson.* Retrieved from https://www.pearson.com/us/higher-education/program/Gregory-Psychological-Testing-History-Principles-and-Applications-7th-Edition/PGM332874.html

House of Lords member Baroness Nicholson brands trans children as sexual predators. (2020). *Trans-Scribe.* Retrieved from https://trans-scribe.blogspot.com/2020/05/house-of-lords-member-baroness.html

Hepp, U., Kraemer, B., Schnyder, U., Miller, N. & Delsignore, A. (2005). Psychiatric comorbidity in gender identity disorder. *Journal of Psychosomatic Research*, 58(3), 259–61. Retrieved from https://www.ncbi.nlm.nih.gov/pubmed/15865950

Jung, C.G. (1970). *The structure and dynamics of the psyche* (Collected works of C.G. Jung) (Vol. 8). Princeton, NJ: Princeton University Press.

Park, S., Lee, Y., Youn, T., Kim, B., Park, J., Kim, H., Lee, H. & Hong, J. (2018). Association between level of suicide risk, characteristics of suicide attempts, and mental disorders among suicide attempters. *BMCI Public Health.* Retrieved from https://www.ncbi.nlm.nih.gov/pmc/articles/PMC5896087/

Strauss, P., Lin, A., Winter, S., Cook, A., Watson, V. & Toussaint, D.W. (2017). *Trans pathways.* Telethon Kids Institute. Retrieved from https://www.telethonkids.org.au/transpathways

Turban, J. (2017). The American College of Pediatricians is an anti-LGBT group. *Psychology Today.* Retrieved from https://www.psychologytoday.com/au/blog/political-minds/201705/the-american-college-pediatricians-is-anti-lgbt-group

Chapter 11:
Restoring the Will to Live

We are born with self-preservation instincts. Sigmund Freud (1922/2009) framed it as the drive to avoid injury and maximise the chances of survival. In the formulation of psychoanalytical theory, it was one of the two essential instincts that propel human behaviour, the other being the sex instinct. Biologically, the presence of life instincts is innate, robust and pretty much lifelong regardless of culture or race.

Like every biological or biopsychological function, however, the life instincts can be interrupted, damaged, suppressed or deprioritised due to trauma states. Many of those physiological or psychological traumas may not be immediately obvious to the onlooker or seem trivial. To the client, such traumas can be cataclysmic, and at times, remain subdued until triggered in a snowball effect that initiates a complex trauma reaction.

There are incidents in nature where the individual's self-preservation instincts no longer operate or are suspended. When a person becomes fatally ill, as in stage four cancer, is in pain or has sustained some kind of traumatic injury, they may choose to end their life by euthanasia or suicide. In some societies, euthanasia has been sanctioned, but in many, it has not, so the person is left with suicide as the only choice to end their life to stop further physical suffering.

In the Netherlands and Belgium, it is legal for a doctor to grant a patient with mental illness a request to die by lethal injection. Amy De Schutter (Cheng, 2017) was granted permission to end her life after having struggled with mental illness for years, taking an assortment of medications and seeing a psychiatrist. None of it helped her.

In Hindu or Yogic traditions, Mahāsamādhi is the final act of intentionally leaving the body (Blackman, 1997). Many yogic masters have been said to predict the day and time they will die so the death is partly psychosomatic, but in their belief, they are said to have extinguished their karma. Some yogis have simply sat and meditated until death. We cannot call this suicide, but it is a loss of the physical self-preservation instinct, although the yogis believe it is part of their spiritual journey.

There are incidents, called the widowhood effect (Ramadas et al., 2013) when one partner of a decades-long relationship dies and the other dies immediately or very soon after, for no apparent biological reason. The second death can occur within a matter of minutes or hours. Recently, Takotsubo cardiomyopathy (broken-heart syndrome) (Pelliccia et al., 2017) has been identified when a partner is lost and stress causes severe weakening to the heart muscle. High-stress-triggering biological reactions like brain injury, asthma or exacerbation of a chronic illness have also been identified as a preceding element.

Therefore, we cannot say the loss of the self-preservation instinct is simply a matter of psychological disturbance or purely emotional dysregulation. It is clear that acute and chronic stress, shock, trauma and a sense of loss not only cause organic shutdown but also damage in multiple systems of the body. This would include a dramatic reduction in serotonin, endorphins and an increase in cortisol, breathing, disorientation and abnormal brain dysfunction.

The Mental State of Suicidal Ideation

Suicidal ideation is a mental state not a mental illness. To treat people from SGD groups who experience suicidal ideation as mentally ill or having a mental illness is dangerous.

Neither should it be described as a psychotic episode. That only adds more burden to the client's already fragile world journey, which may further push them towards suicide. As we have discussed, there are mentally ill people who experience suicidal ideation short- or long-term as a feature of their illness, but to define suicidal ideation as a mental illness is over-diagnosing and not backed by any evidence.

The emergence of suicidal ideation is a breakdown of coping mechanisms within the personality. Think of it as if a fuse has been tripped due to a power surge so the circuits in the brain are not innately reactivating the will to live as they would normally do each minute of the day.

Many practitioners hope that, with time, the client will experience an automatic reboot and will reconnect themselves to the will to live. Indeed, some clients do experience the automatic reboot after they have attempted suicide. Maybe the client frightened themselves with what they did, which jolted them back to the will to live. As a health professional, however, we cannot wait and be passive. The automatic reboot may never happen, particularly if there have been multiple suicide attempts. To do nothing would be negligence.

Intervention is always the best course of action that raises the likelihood of recovery. The practitioner must also not take over the client's life and infantilise them, unless they are non-compos mentis, for that would be disabling recovery by making the client dependent. Our approach must be to offer the client the help they need but not by forcing them, for that is using the stick, not the carrot. People are drawn to the carrot but recoil from the stick. This is equally true whether the suicidal ideations are the result of a short-term crisis or a feature of a mental illness.

Notably, so many different events and experiences can overcome the suicide crisis and restore the will to live in different clients at different times of their lives, and these may not necessarily be a clinical intervention. It could include the kind act of a stranger, a neighbour's interest in their welfare, reconnecting with old friends, soft, reassuring words from a nurse, the promise to help them with housing from a social worker, finding a counsellor or therapist they can connect with, a psychiatrist who takes time to listen to them, the promise of hormones or surgery or an apology from someone who has abused them.

All of these experiences can and do nurture the person's healing processes as they create human connection, feeding their soul and spirit. Clinical intervention without the elements of warm human connection and kindness are unlikely to help the person reinvigorate their will to live. These actions do not necessarily cost a great deal of time but require undivided attention for the time you spend with the client.

It may often be just one thing that you said that will stay with the client and echo continuously throughout their mind, helping them to restore the will to live and making them more resilient to stress reactions.

When Medical Treatment and Free Expression of Physical Sex and Gender is Not Available

Many clients you may see from SGD groups who have become suicidal will be extremely frustrated about not being able to get the care they need. They may be offered care, but it might be the wrong kind, such as conversion therapy or surgery and hormones that they do not want, which will change their bodies in ways that they consider detrimental.

Intersex people in places where there is little or insufficient social medicine may be experiencing battles simply to stay alive because they cannot afford care. As we have seen in intersex surveys, they are often economically disadvantaged. Poverty will come into play for many who cannot afford to take the private medical route to place their bodies in line with what they believe it should be or to simply be able to function the best it can. Others will experience care being blocked by relatives, parents, spouses, hospitals, healthcare workers, governments or laws or they will be forced to wait years for the care they need immediately.

One of the most controversial areas is often that children from SGD groups, who need to change their bodies or present in a particular gendered way, are told to wait until they are older to get the care they request and make those decisions. This is cruel as it tells them what they are is not worthy, valued or good enough. It is a message of discrimination and as we have seen, this frequently leads to depression and the danger of suicide.

During puberty, if your body is changing in ways that you do not want, horrifies you or is not changing in ways you need, it should be considered a medical emergency and treated immediately. Delays in treatment can result in permanently masculinising or feminising of the young person's body in ways that cannot be rectified later. This may cause the person considerable distress. To tell someone their gender performance is wrong is creating a class system and oppressing that person, damaging them psychologically.

The reality, for some, is that their situation might not change and they are unable to find money to pay for care. They live in oppressive circumstances or regimes under which they are trapped in a less than optimum reality. For these people, part of our work may be to try and get them to accommodate to their circumstances and help them find their best-case scenario. That may include encouraging them to be part of a campaign to change those circumstances.

For those who can escape their difficulties, I advise people to do that as no one has the right to force a person to live an unhealthy and unhappy life. If they live in countries where their life is threatened, encourage them to seek asylum in a country with greater SGD acceptance if possible.

Cheshire (2020) reported how trans people in China bought hormones from Thailand because the Chinese medical system was so oppressive and had long waiting times, which is common throughout the world. Medical tourism is standard all over the globe, with people going to have treatments and surgery in other states, countries and continents. There are, of course, risks with this, as medications from abroad may not always be exactly what they are labelled. Corrective or follow-up surgeries may not be viable when someone has returned to their country after having had surgery aboard.

When treatment is not available in one country or is too expensive, I have always advised people or parents to seek care from other countries. This treatment includes hormones or surgery. Practitioners in other countries will do consultations via telehealth electronic channels. Some practitioners find this controversial, but I have found it highly successful. At the end of the day, our job is to promote the person's wellbeing and preserve their mental health to reduce the risk of suicide. Life is too short to wait for the world, ill-informed people, practitioners and politicians to catch up on human rights. Life is what is happening now, not in some distant future according to other people's restricted and uneducated ideas.

Those Who Regret Transition

Some people regret sex and gender alignment or realignment treatment, both hormonally and surgically. Some intersex people regret having their sex or gender transitioned in a way that they consider was outside their nature, without their permission. This is a reality that we must accept as clinicians and some of those intersex people become suicidal and need our help.

They may be sad, depressed, traumatised, angry or in a state of blaming the clinicians who treated them. The press has sensationalised and given these stories high profiles recently, often with poor fact-checking, mainly to create clickbait, which can add to the client's state of anxiety. In some cases, these clients may have had poor levels of treatment. Clinicians provided sub-optimum care by trying to normalise those intersex people, a form of cissexism.

The client may wish to change their body and gender to what they think will better suit them. We must offer no opinion or judgement on this matter and take the lead from the client. Sometimes detransition will work out and sometimes it will not but consideration must be careful. I have seen cases that have arrived in my clinic who have transitioned as many as three times before they settle on a way they can live.

The major complaint of trans detransitioners is often that treatment was carried out without sufficient psychotherapeutic help or a lack of consultation with the client. Those complaints are frequently valid but as clinicians, we must be careful not to take sides. Instead, we must facilitate the client in the present moment by helping them to restore a will to live in the present time.

I have even witnessed clinicians in different countries taking up extremely aggressive campaigns against other clinicians on the complaints of those clients, but that is not our role. As clinicians who help people recover from suicidal thoughts, we are not lawyers or complaints committees.

These clients may experience long-term distress and battle with who and what their sex and gender should be. What they need is space to have catharsis, consider their options and be listened to with empathy. They are likely to need long-term care, struggle with a sense of having been deceived or feel foolish about the decisions they may have made. Some detransitioners may not be able to accept responsibility for their decision to transition in the first place.

Trans people who regret transition and detransitioned are far more common today as they are speaking out as individuals and a movement. The documentary *The Trans Train* (Engholm,

2019) shows a Scandinavian female who transitioned to male in her teenage years within a national clinic system before later detransitioning. The meteoric rise of young females wanting to transition with no previous indication of cross-sex and/or gender identification is often referred to by the controversial phrase "Rapid Onset Gender Dysphoria".

The problem that arises is that detransitioners say they did not have enough psychotherapy before transition and some clinicians say it is due to large levels of mental illness in trans-identified groups. At the same time, many people transition successfully and trans campaigners often say that the waiting time during transition is too long. So, clinicians can find themselves between the devil and the deep blue sea at times about the level of psychotherapy offered. Delaying transition can give rise to suicide and accusations of transphobia. Those who transition and then detransition can experience suicidation, as can those who do not do well when they have transitioned and have a poor quality of life, wellness and mental health.

Some detransitioners talk about how, on reflection, they were probably trying to get away from eating disorders, childhood sexual abuse, problems with identity or relationships and depression. When they were transitioning, they saw it as a rebirth to reinvent their life. Some also have doubts about transition when they do not pass well or for religious reasons when they become involved with certain faiths.

Others talk about how they had been carried along with the glory stories on the internet about people who transitioned. They thought transition might be the answer to their insecurities and problems. At the time of transition, they may have presented as being absolutely sure that they needed to transition. At the beginning of transition, they may even have been euphoric about their transition, but later they are possessed by doubts and end up regretting transition.

Clinicians are often not being clear with patient groups

about this, failing to tell them that treatment is not an absolute that will relieve all of their problems or even the fact that some people do regret transition. For the massive increase in teenage females seeking to live as males, there may indeed be an element of gender dysphoria that is associated with experiencing female oppression. This can only be explored through psychotherapy; however, overly oppressive analysis can cause more existential confusion and problems than solutions.

Therapy should never stand in the way of those who genuinely need hormone blockers, sex-confirming hormones and surgery to stop their bodies developing in ways that will damage their lives. If you are going into puberty and your body is developing male or female physical characteristics, you do not want to have to live with those characteristics. Hormone blockers at puberty can help stop those changes and should not be withheld, because puberty can be restarted by withdrawal of medication if the adolescent changes their mind.

People regret many things in life including pregnancy, abortion, hysterectomy or vasectomy. Sex and gender transition is no different, but those clients who regret are statistically only a small number of those who transition. We must always keep our clinical procedures under review and resist at all times entering into personal judgement of the client or other clinicians. We have a professional duty to report suspected malpractice but should only ever do so with the client's permission. Such accusations can also subject our own practice to the danger of being sued by other clinics for slander or libel. In these circumstances, unfortunately, the major losers are always the clients themselves when services are suddenly cancelled, leaving whole patient lists without care.

Again, detransitioners are a small fraction of the intersex and trans populations, but they have become visible recently due to internet vlogs and press reports. We must support all people from SGD groups when suicidation arises, encouraging them to seek sufficient psychotherapy and support in both the short and long term. They will need to work through their issues and find self-determination and validation.

Suicide and Exhaustion

Death by suicide is often recorded as a temporary disturbance of the mind due to the idea that only a balanced state of mind will not contemplate suicide. This can, however, be an oversimplification and misunderstanding of the state of the person's mind. It is simply what is recorded when the coroner does not want to investigate further.

Many people who attempt suicide are suffering from exhaustion that disturbs the mind and confuses their logical thinking, depotentiating the person's ability to positively future-pace events. That may be long-term exhaustion due to constant harassment, life stressors and frustration with their circumstances, which can lead to a deep, persistent long-term depression.

It can also be acute sudden-onset exhaustion that creates an immediate state of extreme panic and confusion due to shock, sometimes within a matter of hours. That shock may be due to the client finding out they are intersex, being rejected, bullied, harassed, attacked or refused service when they are in extreme need, which is common for many people from SGD groups.

Benson et al. (2020) propose a three-factor model that leads to exhaustion including "lack of trust", "lack of inherent worth" and "suicidal exhaustion". They insist exhaustion plays a key role in suicide ideation and attempts. We can see in reviewing many reports of people from SGD groups who are attempting or considering suicide that these drivers are directly related to the minority stress and isolation that leads to mental exhaustion.

Herein lies a problem for many practitioners because they are unable to distinguish between innate, long-term depression and minority stress-induced exhaustion. The assumption that the suicidal ideations are due to innate mental illness when they are in fact due to exhaustion from minority stress can be fatal for the client as the client receives the wrong kind of or inadequate help.

Giving a patient antidepressants, anxiolytics or antipsychotics dulls their ability to cognitively process circumstances and think through how they may need to go forward in their life. Many clinicians assist in administering these drugs when what the client actually needs is social support and psychotherapy. I have indeed seen cases where, after a person's suicide, the attending physician said, "Well, I offered them medication but they refused". The clinician, however, did not understand the client's social circumstances or anything about people from SGD groups so they were unable to comprehend what the distressed patient really needed.

The pharmaceutical industry's commandeering of melancholia and exhaustion, relabelling them as depression for commercial gain, means that many clients' needs are misunderstood and not facilitated. Since many practitioners are only trained in pharmacological prescribing for assumed psychopathologies, they fail to fulfil their duties as a doctor (meaning teacher).

In state-supplied medicine, there is also the added problem that practitioners are constantly under pressure to cut costs. In a six- to ten-minute consultation with a patient, giving them medication is far cheaper than an hour of talking to them. In private practice, the dynamics can be reversed where the quality of care tends to be higher because practitioners have more time to pay attention to the patient. This is not always true, however, because some practitioners are offering SGD groups care for which they have little experience. Remember there are far more elements that make up the human experience other than singular pharmacological drugs.

It is wise for clinicians to read around orthomolecular supportive treatments and supportive natural treatments (Greenblatt, 2015). Even low doses of lithium in drinking water have been shown to be equated with low levels of suicide (Ohgami et al., 2013). Micro-dosing Lithium Orotate starting at 10mg and increasing up to 30mg shows promise in lowering the incidence of suicide, mood swing and depression. It is far more preferable to the large, full doses of lithium salts (300mg to over 2000mg) that are prescribed psychiatrically, which can have profound side effects such as kidney, liver and thyroid damage, excessive urination and the "blah" experience where people feel they are living in a bubble. Since orotate has smaller molecules, it gains access to the brain more easily so is more effective at a lower dose and more tolerated by patients.

If the client is not sleeping well, doses of 300 to 500mgs of magnesium (per 50 kilos weight) an hour before sleep increases the depth, length and quality of sleep, allowing the necessary REM amounts of sleep. There is a direct link between poor REM sleep and psychosis.

A herbal mixture including Piscidia piscipula, concentrated Matricaria recutita and Eschscholzia californica can be formulated to assist with sleep (Bone & Mills, 2013). Herbs should not be prepared in alcohol if there is any kind of addiction present. Children should be dosed accordingly, and practitioners always need to use a herbalist, not themselves or amateur prescribers.

For extreme anxiety, herbal mixtures may include Matricaria recutita, Melissa officinalis, Passiflora incarnata and Avena Savita. I do not use Humulus lupulus or Piper methysticum as I find they make the patient too soporific.

When persistent soporific depression is present, herbs such as Hypericum perforatum, Panax ginseng and Valerian officinalis may be indicated.

It is also important in exhaustion, trauma and stress to

use Curcuma longa to reduce brain inflammation. Large cheap bags of Turmeric can be bought from grocery supplies stores. These are usually organic because it grows so profusely on its own and the patient can put a half to full teaspoon a day in a lemon juice salad dressing.

Adding 400mgs of Coenzyme Q10 in the morning can increase cellular function for energy. In clients over 50, adding 300mgs of Nicotinamide riboside chloride in the morning daily can boost energy.

Getting the client to abstain from alcohol and stimulants like coffee or smoking dramatically elevates mood and reduces stress on the liver and the gut, allowing the neurological and hormonal systems to work more effectively.

Treating clients with herbs, supplements and nutrition as well as psychotherapy has huge advantages in that the client retains and increases their full cognitive processes.

There is clear evidence that stressed patients also have a gut/brain co-inflammation cycle due to dysbiosis. Administration of probiotics like Lactobacillus reuteri strains DS 17938, morning and night help restore endorphin and serotonin production and reduces brain inflammation (Rogers et al., 2016).

Supplementing with a B complex is indicated unless there are homocysteine problems. Also 1000mgs of vitamin C orally and, if possible, 5000mgs of liposomal C, reduces oxidative stress, decreasing stress on the body and increasing oxygen flow for brain function. Supplementing this with a high dose of vitamin A (10,000iu) increases the brain-derived neurotrophic factor, which aids brain plasticity, facilitating accelerated psychotherapy. However, caution must be used in pregnancy. Vitamin D 5000iu also helps elevate mood.

Testing for the MTHFR gene variants can throw light on erratic behaviour if there are genetic variants needing supplementation with L-methylfolate. Also, hair mineral analysis can reveal mineral excesses or deficiencies and metal toxicity poisoning that severely affects behaviour, particularly sodium, calcium, zinc, manganese, magnesium, mercury, copper, cadmium and lead.

It has become fashionable for some practitioners to experiment with micro-dosing or full-dosing psychotropics like Lysergic acid (LSD) or Psilocybin (Anderson et al., 2018). While shamanic use of these substances can create life transformations, they are cultural psychological experiences. Using such substances pharmacologically on people with fragile suicidal states, with weakened coping strategy mechanisms, runs the huge risk of psychotic decompression and central personality collapse, creating a heightened level of suicidation. In other words, the proverbial bad trip that causes drug-induced and post drug-induced psychosis.

Sleep alone is insufficient in treating exhaustion, particularly when associated with long-term depression where the client may already be sleeping 10–12 hours a day. Exhaustion has traditionally been treated successfully with convalescence in the community. In an industrialised society, however, where SGD groups can experience extreme poverty and social isolation, convalescence is not always possible and with all treatments, we must meet the client where they are and be mindful of what resources they have available.

As practitioners, we must focus much of our efforts on teaching clients from SGD groups who are suicidal the highest levels of self-care and self-worth they can attain in order to counter minority stress and social rejection. Then we must do all that we can to help them accelerate that learning with as much social and community support as possible. Not all clients have resources so we must tailor treatment according to their ability to engage.

Dread of Life
We have all at times experienced a dread of life, whether it be an upcoming exam, driving test, meeting with a belligerent

relative or fear of something dreadful happening. This is indeed natural, for if we had no fear or caution, we would be reckless and continually stumble into dangerous life situations unprepared. We would not live very long as we would be unable to identify danger.

For most of us, most of the time, that dread of life is only temporary, situational, time- or location-specific and when we come out of those circumstances, the dread goes away. The dread is the stress response that sends us into a fight or flight mode when we are faced by a perceived danger or discomfort. We may choose to fight the circumstances in an attempt to change them, but there may be overwhelming odds that are, at that moment, against that change happening. Yet in self-preservation, we may still continue to try to restore a sense of safety by fighting that battle. The fight is driven by the will to live.

Flight can lead us to withdraw from those circumstances in order to make ourselves safe, like hiding in the cave until the dinosaurs have left and we can continue our journey in relative safety. Again, this is driven by the will to live and preserve or restore a sense of peace. This is by far our most prominent and frequent human strategy to take us out of the stress response, not only personally but also with regard to groups, crowds and societal psychology. We envision a future beyond the dread, devise and execute a strategy to take us to that safe place, and thereby cancel the then redundant stress response. We strive for peace and safety.

When the odds of installing or restoring that sense of safety and peace look bleak, we can move beyond that normal fight or flight response and move to the self-death wish as a quest to escape that immeasurably intense discomfort and stress. Paradoxically, the death self-wish itself becomes an act of self-preservation and a quest to find peace.

When that happens, we move into tunnel vision, editing what we see and hear in order to preserve that overriding self-death wish. We are no longer open to considering better options, for that may threaten the strategy to kill ourselves to take us to the promised delivery of peace that we believe death can offer us. It is like being locked in a speeding car with the brake lines cut and the windows and doors will not open. It seems impossible to turn off the engine and the inevitable eventuality by the greater odds is death. The more we might try to escape, the faster the car goes. There is no perceived rescue plan that leads to life. We may even dread the death, but we have surrendered to it as the next logical occurrence as we see no escape.

For those with an existential sex, gender and even sexuality crisis who experience sex and/or gender dysphoria with no perceived possibility of relief, death can become attractive. If you have a sense that your body does not match who you are or your gender performance is not accepted and even scorned, you may begin to hate yourself. When you do not have the positive support you need, that self-hate gets magnified and compounded and you may not see any way out of the dysphoria but death.

If you have no sense of sex and gender dysphoria but consider yourself sex and/or gender diverse and you suffer negative reinforcement and harassment because of who and what you are, a sense of injustice and minority stress can become overwhelming. You may live in a group, family or society that institutionally oppresses you and blatantly ignores your human rights. You can begin to dread each encounter every day, with others or yourself in the mirror, and may perceive the future with a more foreboding outlook by the minute.

When that oppression and personal, institutional or public harassment is constant and chronic because of your sex and gender difference, with no near promise of abatement, by osmosis you may begin to believe your haters. You can conform to the crowd mentality and see yourself as an abomination developing a dread of life. You go to sleep and get

265

out of bed hearing your own voice covered in shame and guilt. You lose self-esteem and a sense of the right to life. You begin and continue to dread being you.

If you have never had a sense of sex and/or gender dysphoria or diversity, it may seem simply academic for you to understand the depths of despondency that people can sink into when they can no longer see a better future ahead. While you may clinically see the client as anxious, depressed and suicidal, it is important to understand suicidality is not simply a subjective set of unregulated negative emotions. In nearly all cases of minority stress, suicide is a response to a dread of life.

In Lille in Northern France, more than 100 students held a protest and sit-in at the entrance to Fenelon High School after a 17-year-old trans student, Fouad, suicided (Spingler & Charlton, 2020). Classmates said she had recently gone public, informing others she considered herself female and had been summoned to speak to school officials after she had worn a skirt to school. A published recording revealed that she was told categorically by school officials that her behaviour was upsetting other students at school. The school even went to the extent of announcing her death as that of a male student.

Fouad was of North African decent, lived in a shelter and a friend, Annabelle, reported that she had suffered both racial and gender discrimination at the school. Even though there were official policies in place for the school to be more tolerant, accepting and protective of vulnerable students like Fouad, the school had ignored those policies. The compounded minority stress Fouad encountered from some students and the school clearly lead to her dread of life and suicide.

Trust
The research that has been quoted clearly shows that people from SGD groups have a low trust level of practitioners from all health disciplines. Clients can be in a catch-22 situation where

they need the help of those practitioners but do not trust them so they withhold vital medical and psychological information.

Many practitioners have scrupulously helped thousands of clients from SGD groups with a high level of service and empathy. I am reminded of the wonderful surgeon Michel Seghers whom I used to send patients to for surgery in Belgium. They always commented afterwards what a kind man he was and how they felt so cared for. He or a nurse would pick them up at the railway station and take them to the clinic. Sometimes, his wife would bring food into the clinic for the patients. They would tell me it was like going to see a kind uncle. Despite all his wonderful work and lives saved, there were times Seghers was attacked by other clinicians competing in the field.

I also worked with the wonderful and inspirational Sydney endocrinologist and teacher Professor Alfred Steinbeck who practised medicine for 66 years and was still in his office as a 90-year-old helping SGD patients. He was genuine and a genius at putting patients at their ease.

Then there was the little old lady called Helen who I worked with at the Earls Court Citizen's Advice Bureau in the early 1970s in London. Trans women who were taking drugs would come for advice and she would give them cakes and sandwiches to take away with them that she had made the night before and brought into work. Many of those women would later die of overdoses, but they would come to the Bureau to see Helen just as much as to see a counsellor. She made them feel worthy and important with her kindness.

Unfortunately, this is not the information that appears in the press as that would not be clickbait, so the media heavily, persistently and predominately publishes stories of clients' treatment that went wrong or was unethical. This can terrorise clients from SGD groups because they feel they may be going into dangerous, unknown situations. It also reinforces the prejudices of oppressors.

There have indeed been terrible practitioners who have done great harm to patients like the US surgeon Dr. John Ronald Brown who left many patients disfigured and dying (Ciotti, 1999). At times, he practised without a license in Mexico and relied on patients' desperation, labelling himself as a "sex change specialist at a budget price". He operated in garages, hotel rooms and on trains.

Trust today is generally built through internet community reports, but there will always be naysayers who will attack you as a practitioner without proper reason, so you must practise good reputation management. Remember, we are in the age of fake news. That does not mean stay quiet and under the radar about the work you do with clients but the opposite. Publish the good work you do so clients can find you and have already built up some trust by your reputation when you meet.

For people from the SGD communities to trust you when they are faced with suicide, you need to have developed your reputation over time as someone who understands their issues and will be empathic to their situation. As someone who has worked in the community for five decades, I get people ringing me who have been recommended by people I saw before the new client was born. Saving lives is as much a dedication as a profession.

Of course, there will always be clients who will not bond with us for a whole host of reasons we might never know. All clients trusting us is a mathematical impossibility. Client compliance can be a real problem in healthcare regardless of our clinical efforts, skills and diligence. Yet we must continue to put a great deal of effort into creating continuous rapport and building trust in the healthcare relationship.

Countertransference of Joy of Life
At times, life is hard for all of us and our traumas are personal to our own life experiences and journeys. Tolerance to stress

and resilience to life catastrophes is either idiosyncratic to our own personalities, bred into us during childhood, a result of our self-development or part of increased tolerance due to exposure to traumatic incidents.

However, we do not exist in a vacuum and our interactions with others constantly shape and reshape our moment-by-moment experiences, mindsets, memories, cognitive processes and emotional maps. When we carry trauma past the time it ceases to be useful as a learning experience, we damage our emotional maps through which we envision life, relationships and our future perceptions.

Our emotional maps are coloured by many things like personal historical experiences, interactions with others, family and social expectations, poverty, success, acceptability and ability to perceive a positive or negative future. They are not set in stone and provided the person is willing and mentally capable, they can be updated at any time in life. One of the features of suicidality, however, is that the person believes the emotional map they have, at the time of the Thanatos crisis, is the one they will have for the rest of their uncomfortable and terrifying life.

History shows us this is not true. We can see how many people who have experienced sex and/or gender dysphoria or diversity have indeed, despite original adverse circumstances, gone on to experience wonderful lives.

The pioneering computer designer Lyn Conway, who was monumental in the evolution of computer technology, started to transition to female in the late 1960s and was fired from IBM because of her transition. The company feared the danger of negative publicity of employing a transsexual woman. At the time, she was married to a woman with small children and the loss of income meant she was unable to support the family. To add insult to injury, California's Social Services said they would take out a restraining order if she ever attempted to see her children.

In 1969, Conway changed her identity and quickly climbed the corporate ladder as a computer architect at Memorex Corporation and Xerox Palo Alto Research Center (PARC). In 1987, the University of Michigan appointed her Professor of Computer Science and Electrical Engineering and Associate Dean of its engineering school. In 2020, when she was 82 years old, and 52 years after her firing, IBM apologised. Along the way, Conway picked up many engineering accolades and awards from equal rights groups for her work in the trans community (Alicandri, 2020).

In a book on the work of German photographer Marianne Breslauer (Breslauer & Feilchenfeldt, 2021), which shows her pictures of butch women from the 1930s, it is evident that many were affluent and managed to live successfully outside societal norms. This was a time when the German/American singer, actress and film star Marlene Dietrich scandalously paraded around Hollywood dressed in men's suits and kissing women, which only added to her fame, public allure and success.

Dr. Alan L. Hart, an American physician, radiologist, writer and novelist, helped pioneer the use of the X-ray for the detection of tuberculosis. Born in 1890 and registered as female, he was allowed to live and dress as a boy in childhood with his parents supporting his gender expression. As Robert Bamford, he married his wife Inez and married later for a second time. In the 1940s, when synthetic male hormones became available, Bamford was able to masculinise more. He was one of the early trans men to undergo a hysterectomy in 1917 and lived the rest of his life and career as a man. Bamford said, "I am happier having made this change than I have ever been in my life so I am ashamed of nothing" (The Legacy Project, 2020).

The outrageously effeminate gay man Quentin Crisp (1968) who paraded through London's West End in women's clothes, make-up, tinted nails and with dyed hair in the 1920s onwards, was constantly under threat of being arrested or beaten up.

Not only was he rejected by society in general but also by the gay men's community because they were afraid of being associated with him as it may have outed them. Living until 93 years of age as a celebrity in New York, he satirically once told me, then aged in his 70s, "All one really has to do to get one up on one's oppressors is outlive them."

It is the joy of the practitioner that adds to the joy of the client. I tell you this history with joy and pride about those people who experienced difficulties in their lives yet overcame them in their own way to live rewarding lives. None of our lives are perfect, and they do not have to be, but we can tell our clients these histories to help them see there may be light beyond their present difficulties, even in the darkest nights of the tormented soul. It is for you to transfer that joy of life to your clients to give them a sense that there may be a future for them.

The Journey of Hope

Life holds no guarantees and can violently change at any time, such is its impermanent nature. There is no one certain way to absolutely deliver happiness to people who wish to adjust their sex or gender presentation; when clinicians offer certainty, they deliver false hope. Each person must equip themselves to find their own path, sometimes with our assistance and the majority of the time without.

Life can be hard at times when you find yourself being attacked just for being yourself, the sex and gender you are or when you experience barriers that are placed in your way to peace and happiness. We have discussed at length the effects of minority stress upon SGD groups and how that affects the mental health of the clients, sometimes driving them to suicide.

We encounter clients when they have been worn down by life, are the worse for wear and feel disillusioned with themselves, humanity and their prospects. However, if we as clinicians buy into that roadmap of no hope, we are not serving our clients but self-serving our own fear of inadequacy.

> *"People have a hard time letting go of their suffering. Out of*
> *a fear of the unknown, they prefer suffering that is familiar."*
> — Thich Nhat Hanh

The client needs a cheerleader, someone who believes things can get better for them when they cannot see that for themselves. That requires us as healthcare professionals to believe that, even in the darkest of circumstances, light can emerge. It requires hope. Each time we have contact with the client, we must encourage that hope from within them with a smile and words of reassurance, jump-starting the client to see hope in their future.

False hope is when we mystically imply that may happen passively, which it will not. Instead, nudging the client to take small steps to improve their life, task by task, can be manageable for them. Whether that be a mental task or doing something practical to change their circumstances, each is as valid. Hope is a belief in a better future that we can build for ourselves, not what someone else gives to us.

What you may do or say can help spark that hope for the client, but once that client has reignited hope within themselves and reinstated the will to live, they then have to keep it alive and only they can do that.

Teach Your Client to Believe in Their Future.

Time, budgets, locational access, departmental policies, bureaucratic incompetence or roadblocks, procedures, processes and protocols may all be against what we may need to do in the moment to help the suicidal person relight the will to live, and frequently are. In those moments, we must decide who or what has the greater need and how far we are willing to go to rescue the client's hope in their future.

272

As someone working in suicide prevention and rescue, your genuine hope needs to be infectious every moment of your working life. It is the currency that you give to the client as a gift with no strings attached. You need to imprint in their mind, memory and thoughts your belief that things can get better for them. It is the light that Florence Nightingale carried that let people who were suffering know that hope is at hand.

This is what I learnt in hospice care when sitting with clients who were dying from the complication of AIDS in the UK in the 1980s. It was a tool of helping people have a good, peaceful, happy journey. Some of those people lived and regained hope, and some died a peaceful death with the hope of better to come.

For the client from a SGD group who has been suicidal, there may still be many difficulties ahead in navigating life, but if they have hope, that journey may be easier and more bearable to travel.

References

Alicandri, J. (2020). IBM apologizes for firing computer pioneer for being transgender...52 years later. *Forbes*. Retrieved from https://www.forbes.com/sites/jeremyalicandri/2020/11/18/ibm-apologizes-for-firing-computer-pioneer/?sh=1c749f967d59

Anderson, T., Petranker, R., Christopher, A., Rosenbaum, D., Weissman, C., Dinh-Williams, L., Hui, K. & Hapke, E. (2019). Psychedelic microdosing benefits and challenges: an empirical codebook. *Harm Reduction Journal*. Retrieved from https://harmreductionjournal.biomedcentral.com/articles/10.1186/s12954-019-0308-4

Benson, O., Gibson, S., Boden, Z., & Owen, G. (2015). Exhausted without trust and inherent worth: A model of the suicide process based on experiential accounts.

Science Direct. Retrieved from https://www.sciencedi-rect.com/science/article/abs/pii/S0277953616303355

Blackman, S. (1997). *Graceful exits: How great beings die: Death stories of Tibetan, Hindu & Zen masters.* Weatherhill.

Bone, K. & Mills, S. (2013). *Principles and practice of phyto-therapy: Modern herbal medicine.* Church Livingstone.

Breslauer, M. & Feilchenfeldt, C. (2010). *Marianne Breslauer - Fotografien: Fotografien.* Nimbus.

Cheng, M. (2017, October 26). 'What could help me to die?' Doctors clash over euthanasia. *Stat News.* Retrieved from https://www.statnews.com/2017/10/26/euthanasia-mental-illness/

Cheshire, T. (2020). Transgender people in China turning to grey market for hormones. *Sky News.* Retrieved from https://news.sky.com/story/transgender-people-in-china-turning-to-grey-market-for-hormones-12169717

Ciotti, P. (1999, December 15). Why did he cut off that mans' leg? *LA Weekly.* Retrieved from https://www.laweekly.com/why-did-he-cut-off-that-mans-leg/

Crisp, Q. (1968). *The naked civil servant.* Johnathon Cope.

Engholm, A. (Producer). (2019). The trans train [Documentary]. Sveriges Television (SVT). Retrieved from https://www.youtube.com/watch?v=oDV-ZL6-Gu0 and https://www.youtube.com/watch?v=73-mLwWIgwU

Freud, S. (2009). *Beyond the pleasure principle* (1st ed.). Dover Publications. (Original work published 1922)

Greenblatt, J. M. & Brogan L. (2015). *Integrative therapies for depression: redefining models for assessment, treatment and prevention.* CRC Press.

Ohgami, H., Terao, T., Shiotsuki, I., Ishii, N. & Iwata. N. (2018). Lithium levels in drinking water and risk of suicide. *Cambridge University Press*. Retrieved from https://www.cambridge.org/core/journals/the-british-journal-of-psychiatry/article/lithium-levels-in-drinking-water-and-risk-of-suicide/7C18AC894A0141D3D89B27282AF35DB2

Pelliccia, F., Kaski, J., Crea, F. & Camici, P. (2017). Pathophysiology of Takotsubo syndrome. *Circulation*, 135(24), 2426-2441. doi:10.1161/CIRCULATIONAHA.116.027121

Ramadas, S. & Kuttichira, P. (2013). Bereavement leading to death. *Asian Journal of Psychiatry*, 6(2), 184–185. doi:10.1016/j.ajp.2012.09.002.

Rogers, G. B., Keating, D. J., Young, R.L., Wong, M.L., Licinio, J. & Wesselingh, S. (2016). From gut dysbiosis to altered brain function and mental illness: mechanisms and pathways. *Molecular Psychiatry*. Retrieved from https://www.nature.com/articles/mp201650?refcode=STEFANPLM

Spingler, M. & Charlton, A. (2020). French teens protest after transgender classmate's suicide. *Associated Press*. Retrieved from https://apnews.com/article/lille-france-gender-identity-906d49e6da9f932e648b835927beld25

The Legacy Project. (2020). Dr. Alan L. Hart – Nominee. Retrieved from https://legacyprojectchicago.org/person/alan-l-hart

Chapter 12:
Brief Therapy

There are so many pressures on us as clinicians to orientate people back to functionality in the shortest possible time. In the case of suicidation recovery, we have the added pressure of getting the client to recover the will to live fast because they are in a life-threatening situation. They may have little money and are in the precarious position of having the structure of their support systems collapsing, as often occurs when suicide takes over the lives of people from SGD groups.

Although earlier we talked about using CBT or even Dialectical Behaviour Therapy (DBT) in organisational settings, in private practice, individual, proactive solution-focused therapeutic approaches can probably be used faster.

The suicidal client has lost future-pacing, positive imaginary optics. Their short-term time frame is filled with trauma and foreboding, and they are unable to move past experiencing SGD minority stress, resulting in a sense of hopelessness.

For these reasons, Brief Solution Focused Therapy can be formulated to produce the fastest and most resilient results (Ratner et al. 2012). Time in therapy is reduced and the client is learning problem-solving skills. They have forward momentum, outcomes can be clearly identified by the client and achievement of the client's goals can be pegged as validation of their success.

The faster you can move a client towards recovery as a therapist, the more quickly they come out of the suicidal state and re-experience self-agency. For some, it may even be the first time in their life they discover they can have self-agency.

Here I am going to make some suggestions on how you might help the client recover their will to live. They are not exclusive and there are many other ways that you might use from your own training. Since many nurses and social workers as well as therapists are also trained in therapeutic techniques, this also applies to those professions.

So many practitioners are afraid of self-disclosure. They have been taught that self-disclosure is a bad thing and that it takes away objectivity from the clinical process, but I do not find this to be so. As an intersex and trans woman, I bring much life experience to my clinical practice that can be utilised as a teaching tool.

I have lived many of the traumas that a lot of my clients experience and have survived, so why would I not share that? Why would you not share your survival strategies that could be adapted for the client to model?

Metaphor

A thousand and one stories gives us a thousand and one possible endings to a narrative (Burns, 2001). Stories are one of the first learning strategies we experience as children and they offer us templates of how to manoeuvre the world, defeat demons, champion a cause, climb out of ravines, weather a storm, overcome tribulation against all the odds and become a hero. What is beautiful about stories is that the humblest of characters can become the hero of the story. Also, they are hypnotic. The messages they carry can be effective at changing the unconscious topography of the mind, thoughts and behaviour in and out of the client's conscious awareness.

As a therapist and during any therapeutic encounter, I tell several stories that can induce somnambulistic trance, bypassing conscious resistance, directly appealing to the unconscious, and initiating rapid psychodynamic change. All are designed to guide the client to a hopeful ending.

Example:

You know when I was very young maybe nine years old (implied vulnerability)...which was a long long time ago (engaging the client's imagination and taking them out of the present time frame, inducing trance)...I lived in very difficult circumstances both my parents had mental health issues and we were very poor (creating rapport by matching distressful circumstances)...we only had three books in the house (identifying lack of resources)...I had this thing going on with my body that I did not masculinise well but everyone insisted on bringing me up as a boy (I too have known some of your difficulty, building rapport)...I hated it and was so unhappy (you are not alone, you have allies)... one day at school the teacher read the class the story of The Wind in The Willows *(engrossment of attention and inducing deeper trance)...do you know it (interrogative engagement)... it is about all sorts of creatures who live on the riverbank and have adventures (creatures who are different can have adventures)...my favourite character was Mr Toad who got into all sorts of trouble (you can be liked and valued even if you are in trouble or are different)...he would have cars...boats...airplanes and have a whole host of catastrophes (it's normal to have catastrophes, you are not bad or wrong, acceptance)... and he would always seem to survive...he'd come home to his friends and tell tales of his adventures (acceptance and overcoming difficulties)...I found them such exciting stories as I listened with wide eyes and could not wait for the next one (reinitiating the will to survive)...I thought "Well, if Mr Toad could have adventures and find his way forward in life so could I" (double narrative) (nested loops (story within a story) (compound suggestion for climbing out of the ravine) the other day I saw a self-righting motorbike that can't fall over because it has gyroscopes that keeps it upright all the time (confusion by changing narrative, call for the ego to rebalance, automatically creating resilience)...Can you imagine no matter how rough the terrain is it can't fall over (interrogative suggestion for resilience)...I bet Mr Toad would like one of those I know I would (double narrative suggestion for resources to cope with life's adventures)...Of course it was only when I was 15 that I could live as female but all that time I remembered Mr Toad was never beaten by his misadventures (modelling survival)...of course it turned out I had just as many adventures as Mr Toad in the end (championing over tribulations)...you of course can survive finding your way forward and have adventures too (direct suggestion)...can't you (testing the change)*

Therapeutic Safe Space

1. Create a safe space in which the client can feel unthreatened. That may need to be away from any aspect associated with the suicide attempt or where those thoughts take place (disconnecting locational triggers).
2. A safe space is a place where no judgement takes place and anyone in that space is protected (establishing their right to dignity).
3. Tell the client it is a safe space in which they are safe and respected and continue to tell them it is a safe space throughout the communication (repetitive suggestion that there is somewhere they can be safe).
4. Get the client to confirm it is a safe space for them and if the response is they do not feel safe, ask them what you both need to do so it is a safe space for them (seeking co-operation and then allowing the client to lead).
5. The most essential part of helping the person is to build rapport and maintain it at all costs. Do not at any time display sympathy for anything the client is experiencing

(empathy allows the client to do the work required and model you, but sympathy makes you look condescending and breaks rapport, making them dependent).

6. For any psychotherapeutic techniques you use which require clients to take follow-up actions, those instructions must be written down for the clients to take away and be easy to understand so there is no confusion.

7. Teach the client the simple 3 Step WOC Suicide Prevention Rescue Drill. You must rehearse them in doing that drill. It needs to be largely in their main representational communication modality and you need to give it to them on a printed sheet.

Simplifying Information and Installing the WOC Suicide Prevention Drill

When someone is in a suicidal or post-attempted suicidal state, they are not thinking rationally but have moved primarily to internal kinaesthetic emotional processing. They have gone through and are probably still in emotional overload. Their information ingestion, sorting and organisational mental strategies will not be operating well and they will often experience cognitive disorganisation and mind fog.

When information is delivered to them, it must be in a simple and sequential form that is easy to follow. If you deliver too much information at once, they will dissociate, shut down external sensory monitoring and be unable to digest that information, offering resistance to suggestions. They will become intimidated.

Leading them into a complex analytical analysis of what has happened will cause them to disengage and they will find such enquiries intrusive and overbearing. Since suicide is driven by negative internal emotional responses, the place you have to meet the client is in the sensory system they are presently using, particularly with the use of your linguistic predicates with regard to sensory experience.

Withdraw from danger: No matter how you are proceeding towards suicide, withdrawal takes you instantly away from of the suicide.

Out of the situation: Making yourself and others safe. Step away from the chair and the noose, puts the pills back in the bottle or down the toilet, steps down from the bridge, etc.

Call for help: Pick up the phone and call your emergency contact, helpline, staff member of the rescue team, a recovery buddy or relative.

Withdraw
Out
Call

Since the reasons for someone becoming suicidal are multiple and complex, it may not be possible to completely change the client in one session. You will need to grade the suicide risk and organise the sessions according to the risk. If you see the client immediately after a suicide attempt and they have funding, you need to see them at least twice a week, eventually reducing to once a week. If you are working in a residential program, I suggest every day.

Experienced therapists can work with people in trauma very quickly, largely using brief solution-focused behavioural therapy and emotive motivational techniques. Therapy must be focused on the client having control of their thoughts, behaviours and emotions and not simply sitting around talking about how the client feels. They know how they feel because they felt like committing suicide.

CBT methods alone, however, without emotional drivers, do not generally move the psyche with everyone because change requires more than cognitive engagement. Therefore, it is up to the therapist to test their methodologies to see what the client reacts to and what makes them most suggestible and susceptible to change.

Meet them initially by matching how they must have felt: terrible, lonely, desperate and unhappy. Acknowledge their distress but then you must move on quickly, leading them into another sensory system to break the state. Using external auditory and internal visual imaginary cues to rehearse WOC is an excellent exercise to break state. Rehearse this so it sets up a Pavlovian response that the client begins to operate in the future when they move towards suicide to break the suicide state.

Example:

> *Okay Roger there is this really neat process I want to teach you (indicating you are prepared to share something valuable and they are worth sharing it with)...you okay with that (interrogative suggestion for eliciting cooperation)... humour me (adding a little levity, exposing that you are vulnerable too, giving some space for resistance)...you know it has helped a lot of people and Dr Tracie O'Keefe who is intersex and trans talks about it all the time (validating the process and indicating it may be applicable to for them)... it's sooo...simple and quick (making the process unintimidating and immediately available)...all you need to do when suicide creeps in is say...**WOC**...in your head and follow the instructions (easy, simple, available solutions are appealing to distressed people)...just three letters...**W**...**O**...**C**... (three-lettered acronyms are easily remembered and lead to association with the process—it becomes an ABC process)... **W** for withdraw from the danger (letter association)...**O** for get out of the situation (direct command to step away)...**C** for call for help (seeking third-party intervention)...so let's rehearse it together (modelling)*

In teaching the client, rehearse them in the process over and over again, give it to them printed out and in big letters to stick on the fridge and send it to their mobile communication device.

Disconnecting Triggers

We are all triggered by so many cues in our day. Those cues can be in any of the five sensory systems (modalities): sight, sound, feeling, smell, taste; and via external (e) sensing or internal (i) sensing as psycho-imaginary experiences. Those triggers may be recently installed or have been established decades ago or in childhood.

Clients will generally know the triggers that plunge them into the suicidal state. They may be experts in what those triggers are, and it is necessary for you to get the client to identify those triggers so they can be aware that they are happening. It is important for you to know those triggers and for the people around them to know what triggers the person to change to the suicidal state.

There may, of course, be complex, compounded multiple triggers, with one triggering another. Many people from SGD groups carry complex trauma due to their life experiences, such as unwanted medical procedures, absence of medical help or abuse. Many may have been brought up in care or have lived on the streets where life was stressful and difficult for them. They often do not disclose the origin of those triggers to clinicians. So, at times, we are working in the dark in getting the client to create light.

The triggers can be locational, certain people, circumstances, words, phrases, partners, family members, catching sight of themselves in the mirror, looking at their body, having to dress a certain way, the way they are forced to present in public, not passing in public, unkind comments, bullying, assault, poverty, media reports, trolls on the internet, being alone, being in the company of others, thinking of their circumstances, fear, despondency, depression and more.

Working in a solution-focused way gets the client to identify what they could do to be safe when they encounter a trigger, because they will encounter those triggers at some stage. Rehearse what they can do not to be affected by those triggers so the triggers are disconnected. They need what is called a pattern interrupter to break the reaction.

trigger > old response > onset of suicidal thoughts (out of control negative thoughts and emotions) > commencement of suicidal thoughts and actions

We used the WOC 3 step suicide rescue drill to interrupt the suicidal thoughts and actions once suicidal thoughts have commenced, installing an interrupter mechanism that interrupts the trigger that happens before the suicide response. The equation we now want is:

old trigger > new response of do something different (break state) > thoughts of coping well > operating their coping skills (creating positive emotions)

The "do something different" can be anything, but it must always be positive and empowering. It can be changing their circumstances, interpreting words and phrases differently, asking a partner to change their behaviour, taking no notice of negative comments from family members, changing location, change to them seeing themselves in the mirror as a superhero, insisting on dressing the way that is right for them within appropriate guidelines, accepting the fullness of themselves as the person they are (and not just their physical self), interpreting unkind comments as ignorance, avoiding bullying and violent situations by changing location, turning off the computer, thinking how they can improve their circumstances and having a project to make that happen, keeping a gratitude journal or focusing on the positive. You are teaching the client to reframe the trigger, which discounts negativity and reframes it as a signal to do things that help them.

As much as you can, get the client to identify the new interrupter pattern of doing something different that stops the suicidal thoughts as it empowers them. Also, it allows them to choose strategies that are realistic in their world. Let it be their great solution and ego-strengthening of their ability to operate it in a problem-solving way. Congratulate them and compliment them on their solutions. Only when they are extremely traumatised with reduced cognitive ability do you suggest the pattern interrupters yourself. However, you can use indirect suggestion to guide them in that direction, and if the client is completely disoriented use direct suggestion.

Example:

So Daisy you tell me that when you were trolled on the internet you felt like killing yourself (identifying the old trigger)... that must have been awful for you (creating empathy by acknowledge distress)...some people really do act stupidly with their privilege...(dissolving guilt and shame by shifting responsibility for those actions away from the client—beginning to disconnect the trigger)...don't they (interrogative suggestion for distancing them from their abusers)...you know there are a few websites that say I'm great and others that say I'm rubbish...imagine my surprise when I read them (giving examples of misinformation)...I wrote to one of them once but never heard back so I just laughed when I read it again...(giving examples of disconnection from a trigger by doing something different)...what do you think you might do when you encounter misinformation (requesting a change of strategy)... block them...yes that sounds good (encouraging generative change)...ignore them and carry on with your day, that's good too (ego strengthening)...you see many people have opinions that are different from our own and sometimes those opinions are based on ignorance...have you noticed that (integrative suggestion for a different frame on other people's ignorance)... they might never get to know what you know and your job is not to be re-educating everyone on the internet because that would be mathematically impossible (validating not responding to trolls)...now there will always be people who will think I'm great and others who think I'm rubbish but it does not keep me awake at night (metaphor for not having to engage with everyone)...and there are lots of people who would like to engage with you in a positive...friendly way so focus on those people (direct suggestion for change of focused attention)... and in the future when you encounter trolls do what you said you could do and focus on the good parts of the day...is that okay...(interrogative test for change, always test the work)... I'm not saying don't go on the net because you will (allowing license not to be contained)...I'm saying be discerning about the communications you engage with just like you have been doing in the past at times (eliciting existing resources)...and focus on the good ones...creating good ones for others too (eliciting altruism can dissolves self-victimisation)...and just think how annoying would that be to trolls (humour).

The Use of Brief Solution-Focused Therapy

Suicidality is an emergency and must be treated intensely, acutely and fast. The client does not have the luxury of extensive discourse or protracted consideration. It is often assumed that most suicide attempts are not serious but cries for help and that the client will naturally get past that point in their life as circumstances change. This, however, is purely an existential perspective and does not consider the difficulties of the everyday lives that many people from SGD groups experience.

Brief solution-focused therapy emerged from Milton Erickson's work and offers us a way to help clients handle their reality and focus on how they can best move forward in their life (Rosen, 1991). Erickson was a pragmatist and would use whatever levers he detected to operate the client's drivers. Paradoxically, he would repackage problems and symptoms as solutions, thereby overcoming resistance.

While the client's options to resolve their sex and gender issues may be limited, life itself does not offer only limited options. As Einstein said:

> *Imagination is more important than knowledge. For knowledge is limited, whereas imagination embraces the entire world, stimulating progress, giving birth to evolution (Viereck, 1926).*

The suicidal person has been struggling with their reality, what they know or do not know, and have seen the future as limited to the extent that they can see no way forward for themselves. Imagination knows no bounds and is creative. In solution-focused therapy, the client is invited to imagine what would be a good way for them to go forward. It is an invitation for them to start problem-solving once again and continue to problem-solve.

Because brief therapy demands the client is involved in interactively creating their solutions, by its very inception, the client is already problem-solving right from the outset. In suicidality, we need to move fast to take the client out of the death-wish and towards working on the will to live.

Example:

> *Just let me say you must have been be exhausted by all those suicidal feelings (rendering suicide redundant as a*

solution)...you must be ready for some peaceful living (raising the possibility of a better life experience)...I wonder what memories you have of feeling peaceful and how you did that (memory recall for good emotional experiences and stating that they have the ability to create them)...it does not matter what you were doing then, only that you were really good at being peaceful (scanning memories for emotional regulation skills)...like learning to ride a bicycle you can remember those skills at any time (conflating the association of riding a bicycle with travelling well emotionally)... you always remember how to do those things (affirming the client's ability to emotionally regulate and direct suggestion to emotionally regulate)...remember when we sat and just breathed earlier how good you were with that (acknowledging competence and breaking the fight and flight state)...well just for a moment (chunking down to make the task easier)...I want you to imagine how you will be as you move into being resourceful again now managing your life (future pacing)... what do you look like (internal visual construction of competence)...keep breathing very slowly now (bring the client back to the calm state where cognitive process can engage)...what good things do you say to yourself inside your head (internal auditory construction of competence)...where does that good feeling in your body begin (emotional regulation)...where does it spread to next (fractionation)...wow you're strong aren't you (interrogative suggestion)...smart aren't you (interrogative suggestion and strengthening ego regulation) ...you're a clever cookie how fast you are working well (acknowledging competence to manage their life and accelerating recovery).

In the script above, you see how we operate in what I call "mind mechanics". We use suggestion in two major sensory systems—sight and sound—and build suggestions for positive internal emotional motivation on top of them.

While we can give tools, we must be careful of giving a prescriptive formula for the client's solutions, because if they fail, it can affirm their perceived self-incompetence and inability to carry on living. Our job is to help the client break the negative emotional state, come out of fight and flight, and reinitiate their solution-focused problem-solving skills. Since many people from SGD groups struggle economically, brief therapy enables us to work quickly with processes rather than content, to help the client kick-start their will to live.

Acknowledging the Dark Side

As human beings, we are not computerised algorithms that simply respond to a CBT new mathematical program because it looks good on paper. Jung (2014) talked about the many different aspects of our personalities and how each archetype serves a purpose. One of those aspects is the dark side that haunts us all. It is the sub-personality that might fill us with self-doubt and fear, give us nightmares and may even have primal psychopathic components that house the Thanatos drive.

Always trying to guide the client away from or to ignore the dark side does not disconnect it or bury its messages to the conscious mind. It acutely demonises the dark side and therefore demonises part of the client, adding to the guilt and shame around being from a SGD group or having suicidal thoughts. The dark side has a job to do to make the whole of the personality work, so it will be persistent until it has the person's attention.

The dark side's voices can say, "You're a freak", "You will never be happy", "The neighbours were right, you should move", "No one will love you.", "Who will accept you as you can't have children?", "You really embarrass your family", "Who would employ you?", "Society will never accept you", "Things will never get better for you", "You might as well just get it over with and kill yourself".

Holmes (2011) talks about how working with and negotiating with all sub-personalities can help restore ego control and psychodynamic balance. The life force we experience means that the majority of our sub-personalities want us to live. Simply trying to contain the dark side is like trying to stop a runaway train.

These dark suicidal messages bring strong emotional negative feelings and self-doubt. The internal kinaesthetic negative force does not react solely to logical analysis. It persists in the face of logic. As Ford (2009) says, you need to talk to your shadow side sub-personality and respect it as part of the whole of you.

Example:

I've just got to say to you that so many people have these thoughts (helping the client recognise that they are not alone and not the only one to run away from the dark side)... in fact I've had some of them myself in one form or another (compounding rapport)...Oh and sometimes they are terrifying when they arrive (acknowledging the person's fear)... it's your dark side talking to you...you know (acknowledging the shadow side)... and we might naturally want to run away from it but the faster we run the faster it runs (mirroring the client's experience—pacing)...just imagine for a moment that you stopped running and listened to what it had to say (taking the person out of the flight response)...in fact just have a conversation with your dark side (putting the central managing personality on an equal footing with the dark side)...ask it "What are you trying to tell me?" (putting the central managing personality back in control)...does what it's saying make sense and does it have a point (listening not running)...it wants you to kill you...mmm...well that's a bit extreme isn't it...because if you died it would die (reframing the death-wish)...does it have any other information that

might help all of the other parts of you (holding the dark
side to standard of evidence)...it does not think you have
any prospects in life (dialogue between subpersonalities)...
Oh does it have any solutions other than killing yourself...
(solution creation)...no...Okay, does any other part of you
have any solutions (multiple option creation)...Ah, one part
of you says change your circumstances (acknowledging
the possibility of change)...another part thinks you need to
hang out with people who might be similar to you (the client
reinitiating the will to live)...that sounds good I like that
one...you're getting good at this (ego building)...well put your
arms around that dark part hug it and thank it for kicking
off the debate of what to do next (demythologising the dark
side)...I'm excited for you that you are stopping running and
creating more possibilities...really well done, keep going (sug-
gestion for continuing the solution-focused thinking process)

Wiping and Reprinting

Suicidal people run negative thought loops around and around
inside their mind as obsessive-compulsive thought patterns.
They are largely focused on the negative and, at times, the
invitation of death can offer a perceived positive benefit that
they will not suffer anymore. The negative thought loops are
traumatising and retraumatising. Each time they are experienced and recoded in the mind they blow the trauma up in size
to be more traumatising as the person moves towards suicide.

In hypnotic terms, we call this fractionation. It is taking
an experience and increasing it each time we re-experience, a
form of magnification. It is more intense because we are familiar with the experience and have practised it, magnifying the
intensity of the experience by self-suggestion. Repetitive self-
suggestion creates neural pathways in the brain that induce
automatic thought, behavioural and emotional patterns.

Whether they are negative or positive is relevant because they either create or disturb hedonic balance (Lindquist et al., 2016), which is our neurological perception of right or wrong. What we know from CT scans is that trauma and extended exposure to stress can shrink the brain, scar it and change its structure (Bremner, 2006).

However, what we also know is that hypnosis, meditation, visualisation, prayer and skilful psychotherapy can remodel the brain and also very quickly create a neurological adaptive workaround. Studies of brain plasticity (Cramer et al., 2011) show us that its structure changes according to extrinsic and intrinsic stimulation which would include experiential interactions. This means all those internal experiences of imagination, psychotherapy and psychodynamic change can repattern neuronal activity, thoughts, behaviours and emotions, as we see quickly in brief solution-focused therapy. So, we can literally wipe the prevalence of trauma effects in the brain by wiping and re-patterning memories.

There are different techniques for wiping experiences from conscious awareness and in extreme trauma recoding them differently so that desensitisation takes place. We are also installing substitution experiences with dialectical behavioural therapy (McKay, 2019), tapping (Stapleton, 2019), eye movement desensitisation and reprogramming (EMDR) (Shapiro, 2018), time line therapy (James & Woodsmall, 2017), Milton Erickson's memory supplementation and pseudo orientation in time (Erickson & Rossi, 2009), narrative therapy (Denborough, 2014), hypnotical-induced amnesia and hypermnesia and hypnotic direct suggestion for experiential supplementation (Rossi et al., 2016).

Therapy, when it is done well, is a process of editing, reimprinting and recoding thoughts, behaviours, language (both internal and spoken), actions, values and emotions. We are helping people change their story. The only use for old stories is the good experiences and lessons you can learn when you remember them. Any positive constructive lessons you learn could be useful in the future. To alleviate anxiety and trauma, we must change the old story and recode those changes in order so our experience in the present can be fruitful.

Reisner et al. (2016) in dealing with PTSD-associated sex and gender dysphoria in a community-based study found an elevated risk of mental health problems in transgender persons who experienced discrimination.

When we read many autobiographical accounts of the lives of people from SGD groups, they frequently contain accounts of historical trauma. These traumas can include having undergone unwanted, involuntary surgeries, lack of available medical help and social support, sex and/or gender dysphoria, rejection by families, bullying, social and workplace exclusion, harassment, violence and poverty.

Many of our clients describe some kind of life traumas that they still carry with them and are constantly re-exposed to due to PTSD. Those traumas can be directly related to their sex and gender experiences. When the sex and gender issues have not been resolved, the client can stay in the trauma state as a form of self-defence, either consciously or unconsciously. They may appear hostile, distressed, disturbed or even paranoid, but they are actually constantly re-experiencing those traumas, particularly when they become suicidal.

Often clinicians do not understand the extent of the impact of those traumas on the client's mental health and wellbeing, so the PTSD is missed during assessment. The person is incorrectly pathologised with mental illnesses as the reason for suicidal ideations. So, it is paramount that clinicians screen for PTSD associated with sex and gender diversity in all people from SGD groups who experience suicidation.

When a diagnosis of PTSD is in fact recognised in these clients, constant support may be needed over the short-term to de-escalate the suicide risk. Here, again, we run into the resources and funding problem in that how much care we are able to offer the clients. There may or may not be medical expertise and funding available to resolve unwanted sex difference or provide surgeries, hormones or medications. We may also not be able to offer the remedy of changing other people's attitudes towards the client unless that involves family therapy or co-ordination with schools and workplaces.

So, we are often left with the task of helping the client deal with their perceptions of their imperfect and non-ideal life and helping them move beyond past traumas. If this does not happen, it is likely that the PTSD trigger that initiated suicidal ideation will produce repeated effects and suicide attempts.

So, I strongly propose we screen for PTSD in every client from SGD groups who encounters suicidation; and posit not to do so would be negligent. Again I suggest that not only is it possible that PTSD could be or probably is present, but in fact, it would be surprising if it were not in some form or another.

Treating that SGD-related PTSD requires the clinician to be wholly familiar with the circumstances that installed the original triggers in the first place. This is why in this text I have taken extensive care to expose the reader to the world that SGD groups live in and the difficulties they encounter in their everyday lives. There are no shortcuts here because if you do not understand the circumstances of the original trigger and are unfamiliar with the medical and social background issues, it is highly likely that the client will see you as patronising, incompetent and uninformed, thereby breaking rapport. The last thing that the suicidal person wants to have to do is to teach you the 123s of sex and gender diversity.

A dangerous assumption can be that the PTSD was the cause of the sex and gender dysphoria or diversity. That has frequently been propagated by theorists who have difficulty accepting that diversity is part of nature, not solely the result of trauma. This was portrayed in films like *Psycho* (1960) and has been re-themed in many other films. Even though clinicians or theorists may be people of science, many are creationists tethered to "Adam And Eve" philosophies.

Trying to quell suicidality by assuming trauma or a lack of mental development caused the sex and gender diversity is nothing less than reparative therapy, which research clearly shows us is harmful. Wright et al. (2018), in a systemic review, found no evidence of reparative therapy effectiveness but did find harm from such treatment. It attacks the client's existing coping mechanisms and in suicidality runs the risk of causing a complete psychotic breakdown.

The way to go is to support the client's journey of self-discovery.

Example:

Gosh Bobbie I can see you have been struggling (acknowledging the client's pain and placing it in the past)...and my heart goes out to you (validating that they are worth caring about and anchoring safety and respect)...I want you to know that I can't imagine that pain because I'm not you and have not travelled your journey (acknowledging what they are experiencing is real to them)...I was wondering what was setting you off into suicidal thoughts (allowing them to tell their story)...Gee that must have been tough for you and I see how it might have looked frightened (changing linguistic sensory modality to break the kinaesthetic state (visual scrambling also time shifts experience by putting fear into the past tense)...I hear what you are saying and if I were you I might have thought the same (empathy building rapport)... maybe...just maybe...you can rethink the voices in your head (further changing to auditory linguistic sensory modality to break the kinaesthetic state (auditory scrambling) including the possibility of different kind of internal dialogue) indirect suggestion)...you know when I get haunted by the past I often say to myself, "Damn it, that's not going to get the better of me—buzz off" (inviting the client to model you)...just try that...in fact sometimes I get quite angry with the past and say to it "How dare you follow me around" (channelling anger and redirecting it takes people out of apathy and directs their self-anger to a tangible metaphorical concept—the past)...I wonder if you might like to tell your past off for following you around...give it a good talking to (disconnecting the client from their traumatic past)...you might think it a bit odd but it really makes me feel better (catharsis)...just give it a try now inside your mind for a moment...I know sometimes life is not fair and I know sometimes life can be a rotten stink bag and you want good times—give the past the sack (acknowledging the suicidal instinct and separating the client from the traumatic life—Erickson's apposition of opposition)...so think about sacking the old life and the stuff that went before (indirect suggestion for separating from past traumatic trigger)...whatever it was it is no more (bring the client into the present time frame)...now is time to begin again and see how you can make it taste sweeter (we are working in five sensory systems and using linguistic modalities to bring the client into the present and separate them from their PTSD emotionally-driven triggers from the past)...what will it look like in the future as you learn to feel good (psychoimaginary visual future pacing, giving power to the client to create the future)...it won't always be easy...in fact sometimes it will be hard (reality testing)...but step by step...second by second...minute by minute...put one foot in front of the other (chunking and progressive attainment)... what will you be saying to yourself as you get stronger now (psychoimaginary auditory future pacing)...maybe you can own your body and work out how to go forward together (psychoimaginary kinaesthetic negotiations)...you will make it better (direct suggestion)...I don't know how you will go forward...but I do know it can taste sweeter as you do that (psychoimaginary gustatory future pacing)...nothing smells better than success (psychoimaginary olfactory future pacing)...you are valid for who and what you are (teaching self-validation)...your journey is valid...there will be good times (future pacing positive internal emotions, giving hope)...you will make that happen in a way that is right for you (direct command suggestion)

We cannot help the client solve all of their problems at once. Suicide rescue is about bringing the client into a resourceful place in the present so they can then begin to deal with their life situation.

The Hero's Journey

Suicidal people are not their own heroes but their own perceived failures, particularly for many people from SGD groups. They can carry intergenerational trauma and social oppression around in their psyche that shades their view of themselves. It is hard to create or maintain your own good self-image and self-esteem when you are constantly besieged with personal and public attacks on who and what you are or maybe striving to become.

The client may have little knowledge of the history of SGD groups, grown up in an isolated community or been told that they are wrong, so they have no idea of their hero within. They may never have heard of Casimir Pulaski, Georgina Turtle, Bonnie Hart, Tiger Devore, Lady Colin Campbell, Sally Gross, Caster Semenya, Chevalier d'Éon, Reed Erickson, Christine Jorgenson, Kate Bornstein, Jamison Green, Stephen Whittle, Jin Xing, Laxmi Narayan Tripathi, Dominique Jackson, Janet Mock, Christie Elan-Cane, Norrie May-Welby, Ru Paul or Quentin Crisp.

They may not know of those people from SGD groups who stood up and were counted. If they have no knowledge of the SGD heroes, they may not have hope for their life and have little to reach for during their own journey.

The hero's journey, while inspired by others, is a personal journey for the client. It is the quest to ascend beyond the suicidal crisis that they have encountered. For that journey to be inspired, it requires the health worker helping them to truly believe in that journey and the ability of the client to make that journey to become their own hero by embracing their diversity.

Here we are not talking about wealth, success, fame, beauty and all the things the media exalt as success but about the overcoming of everyday life struggles and challenges, the transcendence over adversity against all the odds, including the threat of suicide.

This is not the health worker making the journey for the client or pushing them to do so but instead teaching them to make it themselves, one foot in front of the other.

Example:

> *Can I tell you a story (not an interrogative statement but an announcement that I am going to share something important) ...I'm a bit of domestic body at home (beginning the story with a quite mundane statement)...I'll methodically do the laundry, take care of our apartment...I don't cook every day in fact not very often...my life is quite ordinary in many ways (making you ordinary so you both start on an equal footing)... there is one thing I did years ago however that turned me into a superhero...I started to make banana and strawberry ice-cream (ordinary to point of boredom so the client goes into a trance)...my partner went wild over it...loved it...has to have it every day and I have been living off the glory of that introduction ever since...I became the ice-cream superhero even when*

I am not the one making it (making the journey to being a superhero accessible)...we can all get from day to day with our triumphs...no matter how small or large (associating small triumphs and large achievements)...in fact getting from one day to the next is a hero's journey that we all make and I want you to celebrate that for you (making the client a success)... and we can look for our triumphs along the way (enlisting the client in the hero's journey)...you're a hero for simply being here today...so celebrate that with me (re-enforcement of their will to live)...what else is there you can imagine that you could do now along your hero's journey that helps you live well (future pacing) indirect suggestion)...and you can have many triumphs (direct suggestion).

Physical Movement

As much as possible, get the client to move their body each and every day by walking and exercising. People in the suicide response have dissociated from their bodies and minds and are essentially checking out of their life. They may even have disassociated from their body because they are experiencing sex or gender dysphoria. When the body is not moving, it is producing less serotonin and endorphins. By getting people to engage physically, we are getting them to re-associate with their body and forcing cognitive engagement.

That might not change any sex or gender dysphoria if it is present, but it will help them get back some control and help them move out of subjectivity because they have to pay attention to manoeuvring and negotiating, which is a distraction from suicidality. If you hate, are angry with, dislike, feel let down by or are ashamed of your body, it may seem a great distance to re-associate back into it. It is, however, the only body a person has, so taking whatever aspect of control over it can help create self-agency and power.

In suggesting this as a health professional, we have to be mindful of how some members of the public react in a hostile way to differently-sexed bodies and gendered experiences. So, we need to guide clients to exercising in safe spaces that are comfortable for them and not pushing them into public spaces that they may find difficult to manoeuvre.

Oral Consumption

With people in trauma, it is not wise to thrust overly dramatic changes on the client all at once; that would overwhelm them. Many people who move to suicide are often in poor health, particularly when drug or alcohol addictions are involved. Gilbert et al. (2018) carried out a systemic review and found increasing evidence of elevated alcohol abuse in transgender and gender minority populations. I have also talked about the plague of drugs and alcohol among people from SGD groups I have encountered.

My own opinion is that addiction is as much a medical emergency as suicide. If a client from a SGD group is suicidal with addiction, I suggest it is paramount to try to get them to address the addiction issues to restore cognitive processes.

As a naturopath, I am always going to suggest a route away from medications wherever possible towards herbs, and supplements, which carry just as much evidence for recovery from depression, anxiety and trauma as does allopathic medicine but typically without the side effects.

In short-term clients, it is not possible to influence diet, but in the long-term, leading them to a low-fat, whole food, plant-based diet will help reduce brain inflammation, decreasing gut dysbiosis and thereby increasing serotonin and endorphins.

The Peaceful Mind

People who are experiencing trauma, depression, anxiety and suicidal ideation do not experience internal peace but are possessed by negative emotional dysregulation, increased cortisol, adrenaline and noradrenaline. This damages the brain, scars the hypothalamus and enlarges the amygdala, reducing cognitive ability and emotional regulation.

The creation of or recreation of peace states takes the client out of the fight or flight response. The brain can begin to rebuild itself, restoring cognitive ability and emotional regulation. How you guide the client to that peace state depends on your skill set and the amenability of the client. If they are religious, pray with them; teach them meditation, self-hypnosis and how to sit in peace in their centred self. Take the lead from the client as to what they are open to experiencing but guide them to more alpha and theta brainwave activities which promote neuroplasticity and the creation of new neural pathways.

The Language You Use

In working in this area every word, intonation and gesture counts. Pragmatically practitioners need to develop a deep knowledge of psycholinguistics and the hypnotics of delivery of meaning, intent and suggestion. Suicide rescue and prevention are time-sensitive so it is vitally important that practitioners' delivery is maximised to induce motivation towards recovery.

For those practitioners not trained in hypnosis or how to deliver somnambulistic conversational hypnotic suggestion, it is a good idea to take a basic hypnosis course to begin to understand the power of suggestion, both indirect or direct.

When people are suicidal, they are invested in their suffering and will defend the right to suffer against perceived inarticulate do-gooders. The art of suggestion surpasses all else to remove unwanted human misery.

Miller and Rollnick (2012) talk about motivational interviewing where they divide communication into three styles —directing, guiding and following, all of which are valid. It is useful for practitioners to be artful in all these styles. Ultimately, however, all therapeutic communication is directive, even when the client generates their own restoration of the will to live.

References

Bremner, J.D. (2006, December 8). Traumatic stress: Effects on the brain. *Dialogues in Clinical Neuroscience.* Retrieved from https://www.ncbi.nlm.nih.gov/pmc/articles/PMC3181836/

Burns, G. (2001). *101 Healing stories: Using metaphors in therapy.* Wiley.

Cramer et al. (2011). Harnessing neuroplasticity for clinical applications. *Brain.* Retrieved from https://pubmed.ncbi.nlm.nih.gov/21482550/

Denborough, D. (2014, January 6). *Retelling the stories of our lives: Everyday narrative therapy to draw inspiration and transform experience.* W. W. Norton & Company.

Erickson, M. & Rossi, E. (2009, March 23). *The February man: Evolving consciousness and identity in hypnotherapy.* Routledge.

Ford, D. (2009). *The secret of the shadow: The power of owning your story.* Harper Collins.

Gilbert, P., Pass, L. Keuroghlian, A., Greenfield, T. & Reisner, S. (2019). Alcohol research with transgender populations: A systematic review and recommendations to strengthen future studies. *Drug and Alcohol Dependence.* Retrieved from https://www.ncbi.nlm.nih.gov/pmc/articles/PMC5911250/

Hitchcock A. (1960). *Psycho* [motion picture]. United States: Paramount Pictures.

Holmes, T. (2011). *Parts work: An illustrated guide to your inner life.* Winged Heart Press.

James, T. & Woodsmall, W. (2017). *Time line therapy: And the basis of personality.* Meta Publications.

Jung, C.D. (2014). *The archetypes and the collective unconscious* (Collected works of C.G. Jung) Kindle Edition (2nd ed.). Routledge.

Lindquist, K., Satpute, A., Wager, T., Weber, J. & Barrett, L. (2016, May 26). The brain basis of positive and negative affect: Evidence from a meta-analysis of the human neuroimaging literature. *Cerebral Cortex.* Retrieved from https://www.ncbi.nlm.nih.gov/pmc/articles/PMC4830281/

McKay, M. (2019). *The dialectical behavior therapy skills workbook: Practical DBT exercises for learning mindfulness, interpersonal effectiveness, emotion regulation, and distress tolerance.* New Harbinger Publications.

Miller, W.R., and Rollnick, S. (2012). *Motivational interviewing: Helping people change.* (3rd edition). Guilford Press.

Ratner, H., George, E. & Iveson, C. (2012). *Solution focused brief therapy: 100 key points and techniques.* Routledge.

Reisner, S., Hughto, J., Gamarel, K, Keuroghlian, A., Mizock, L. & Pachankis, J. (2016). Discriminatory experiences associated with posttraumatic stress disorder symptoms among transgender adults. *Journal of Counseling Psychology*, 63(5), 509–519. Retrieved from https://pubmed.ncbi.nlm.nih.gov/26866637/

Rosen, S. (2009). *My voice will go with you: The teaching tales of Milton Erickson.* W. W. Norton and Company.

Rossi, E., Erickson-Klein, R. & Rossi, K. (2016). *The collected works of Milton H. Erickson*, M.D. The Milton H. Erickson Foundation Press.

Shapiro, F. (2018, February 25). *Eye movement desensitization and reprocessing (EMDR) therapy: Basic principles, protocols, and procedures* (3rd ed.). The Guilford Press.

Stapleton, P. (2019). *Science behind tapping: A proven stress management technique for the mind and body.* Hay House Inc.

Viereck, G.S. (1929, October 26). What life means to Einstein. *The Saturday Evening Post.* Retrieved from https://www.saturdayeveningpost.com/wp-content/uploads/satevepost/what_life_means_to_einstein.pdf

Wright, T., Candy, B. & King, M. (2018). Conversion therapies and access to transition-related healthcare in transgender people: A narrative systematic review. *The BMJ.* Retrieved from https://bmjopen.bmj.com/content/8/12/e022425.full

Chapter 13:
People Who Decided to Live

Here are five cases in which I worked to help people from SGD groups overcome suicide. The patients' identities and names have been changed for confidentiality. I work psychodynamically, behaviourally, emotively, and hypnotically within a solution-focused paradigm.

They are followed by five personal accounts, in people's own words with their real names and all happy to be identified publicly, including my own.

Mathew

A young man, who looked 18, was brought to see me. He turned out to be 31 years of age. He was fresh-faced, tall, thin and willowy, with a slight build. His mother was a former patient of mine whom I saw because she had a neuro-degenerative disorder. He was a virgin and had never had a relationship.

His father was a family doctor and his mother an engineer. There were two other brothers and one sister, all of whom had done well professionally. The family was well off, close and very loving. Mathew had been sent to a private boys' boarding school where he was bullied because he did not fit in with aggressive sports and the roughhousing in which teenage boys create pecking orders. He described his school years as extremely difficult.

He had not done well academically, had poor focus and memory and was dyslexic. Since school, he had worked intermittently as a gardener and had periods of depression.

He had been on and off antidepressants. Although he enjoyed the work, he found it too tiring at times to work full time. He had always lived at home with his parents who had no problems supporting him when he was between jobs.

Two months before I saw Mathew, his family had an endocrinologist as one of the dinner guests. On seeing Mathew and hearing about him, he advised that Mathew be tested for Klinefelter's Syndrome. When the test came back positive, Mathew suddenly became depressed and attempted suicide by swallowing sleeping pills. His mother, extremely worried about his mental state, looked in on him in his bedroom, found him unconscious and rushed him to hospital for a stomach pump.

The father, who was upset about not recognising Mathew's symptoms of Klinefelter's, wanted him sectioned for a 48-hour observation in a closed psychiatric ward. His mother, fervently opposed to such a move, took him home and kept a close eye on him, taking time off work herself. It was four weeks after the attempted suicide that I saw Mathew.

He told me that he saw the diagnosis of Klinefelter's as yet one more burden to carry in life that he thought was too much for him to shoulder. For him, it confirmed that he was the runt of the litter and that his schoolmates were right in that he indeed was weak and defective after all.

He was highly surprised when I disclosed to him that I was intersex and did not see myself as defective at all, although I once did. I asked him to try and begin to see the diagnosis of Klinefelter's as a marvellous blessing. It indeed explained so many things that he had experienced, allowing him to now live his life according to what would be right for him. It could be seen as a great opportunity, like at last understanding why some tomatoes grow and some do not; because different kinds of tomatoes may need different amounts of water or different soil.

Over two weeks, I saw him four times and he agreed to begin testosterone therapy to change his body to more how he had always wanted it to be. He was clear in his identity that he was male and that was not negotiable. The testosterone had dramatic results with him growing facial and body hair. After two years and endless visits to the gym, he considerably increased his body mass to the extent he now passed as an average male, which pleased him enormously. He also entered into a relationship with a woman.

I saw him a few years later for grief counselling after his mother had died. He had no suicidal thoughts, worked part-time and was still in the relationship. Although he had a micropenis, the couple had been creative with sex and neither of them wanted children.

The reframing of Mathew's situation as an opportunity and allowing him to remodel transitioning from him perceiving himself as an intersex victim to self-created champion made his life sustainable and joyful.

Advick

A 29-year-old trans man presented to me. The only female daughter of a middle-class family, he had left India at 18 to study in London. He left behind his mother, father and two brothers and had never returned. During the interim, he had earned a first-class Honours Degree, two Masters, both with distinctions, and was now engaged in a PhD. He had never worked and the family had been sending a modest stipendiary for him to continue his studies.

Advick had a haircut that hid a lot of his face and wore a well-worn man's suit but had not taken hormones or had surgery. He pretty much kept himself to himself, had no friends and tried to move through life without being noticed. He had plaster casts on his right foot and hand.

Recently, the family had been demanding that their daughter return to India to be married to a suitable man the family had found or they would cut off the allowance.

They seemed unaware of how Advick was living. Distraught at the very thought of returning to India and being forced to live as female, he had got drunk and thrown himself out of a second-floor window of the student house he lived in. The landlord, who was British/Indian and lived next door, insisted he seek help to be able to stay in the house.

Advick's number one priority was to continue to live in the UK and transition physically to male. I suggested he approach his professor and ask for teaching work for which he was well qualified. I emphasised how necessary it was to create income to finish the PhD. I told him I would help him transition, but I wanted to see him get practical in his life and become financially independent.

The teaching work took some months to transpire. In the meantime, he had gotten part-time work as a researcher in a law firm that said if they were happy with him, they would sponsor his work visa. Since he had buried his head in his studies for ten years, I gave him the challenge he had most avoided: mixing with others.

The family did indeed cut off the allowance and Advick had to be frugal until the teaching work kicked in and he had two incomes. He started testosterone, was able to save to go back to India for chest surgery without telling the family, got his work visa and was aiming to get into chambers to train as a barrister when he got his PhD. He told me he was far too busy to consider killing himself anymore.

When he asked me how he should disclose to his family, I told him I had absolutely no idea. I was not Indian and did not understand the familial or social dynamics involved. I told him he was smart enough to work it out and to be as kind to them as he possibly could be because they would experience the death of their daughter.

Sex and gender dysphoria was not Advick's greatest problem but the fact that he was infantilised by being economically dependent on his family. His greatest fear was the threat of going back to India to live as female. Creating the ability to work and make money matured his personality, gave him self-agency and the freedom to live as he wished.

Mo

At just-turned 16, Mo presented as androgynous with black nail polish, short cut hair, baseball cap, waistcoat, culottes and boots. The effect was intentional for they identified as gender-neutral or gender non-binary, neither male female. Registered as female at birth and born into a lesbian relationship, with an unknown male sperm donor, they attended a girls' school and had lived in a separatist feminist world as a child, to the exclusion of male figures. Mo was comfortable with the pronouns he or she and him/her/they/them.

Somewhat of a rebel at school, during puberty Mo started to identify as non-gendered, much to the horror of their mother who saw it as a betrayal of feminism. The original lesbian relationship Mo was born into fell apart and the mother had a string of live-in lovers, some that Mo got on with and some they did not. Mo commented that they had always thought of the home as the mother's house and not Mo's home.

Mo was a cutter, with both arms showing dozens of scars from three years of cutting. They were staying with an aunt and female cousin at the time I saw them as relations had become too fractious with their mother. Mo ran away and the school refused to take them back because they were cited as disruptive. A week previously, Mo cut too deep and began to bleed out, needing to be rushed to hospital for surgery. When I asked if they intended to kill themselves, they said they just did not know, maybe.

Mo's extremely high stress levels, acting out and self-destructive harming behaviour showed all the signs of long-term emotional abuse. Mo refused to meet with the mother and received several phone calls from her a day, during which the mother shouted down the telephone at them that it was a phase and Mo should behave like a proper woman now. The aunt reported that after each call, Mo became depressed and started cutting.

Mo said they did not want to be a man at the moment but could not rule that out in the future. Most of all, they never wanted to go back and live with the mother. The aunt had offered for Mo to stay with them until they were 18 and could get some kind of training to make a living.

Mo was confused in the first session that I was not interested in talking about their gender identity but wanted to focus on stopping the self-harming. We agreed they would not take any calls whatsoever from the mother and the only person to speak to the mother would be the aunt. Since they were under the aunt's roof, I considered the aunt the principle guardian for the moment.

We agreed Mo had to keep a cutting diary and every time they cut to write down when, how, for how long and why they cut. Five days later, analysis of the diary showed cutting had mainly become a habit to gain control when they thought they were out of control of a situation, which was pretty much most of the time.

The central part of therapy was teaching Mo to have control over their own life, second by second, minute by minute and day by day. So, I asked Mo to intentionally identify in their daily diary how they wanted control and what would give them control, then to do that again and again. This was the transfer of obsessive-compulsive actions to self-preservation.

We also helped them future-pace a life without trauma. This became possible when no communication with the mother was happening, as she was clearly a source of constant abuse. With no physical, auditory, visual, emotional contact with the mother, and distance from her, this reduced Mo's stress levels, cutting and self-harming. This gave room for self-nurturing to take place in a positive, safe and caring environment that the aunt provided, which eliminated suicidal ideation.

Cutting was an emotional response to stress and removing contact with the mother removed Mo's major stressor. Mo needed to learn to monitor their own thoughts, behaviours and emotional responses to overcome the cutting and suicide possibilities, which also taught them to gain control over their general emotions.

Samantha

This 39-year-old, 15-year post-transition trans woman referred to herself as of trans origin. Working as a fashion buyer, she was not out publicly so she was living stealth with no contact with her family or culture of origin. Work was busy and she had to travel a great deal of the time, which severely restricted her social life. This had, however, allowed her to buy her own apartment and do quite well financially.

Transition had been easy for her in that she found a therapist who readily prescribed hormones and she paid for surgery abroad with no questions asked. She had taken the fast route to transition and avoided any real discussion about what she was going through. The therapist did not challenge that in any way.

The problem that arose for her was, while she passed as female, she had no skills for dating or forming romantic relationships. She was beginning to question transition and having suicidal thoughts, thinking that she may have done the wrong thing that had doomed her to being alone forever. The girl-friends she had were one by one slowly getting married and having children.

We rarely talked about her being trans. Instead, I focused on how many professional women I saw in their late thirties who were not getting married who were really her contemporaries. In her case, because she had been socialised as a boy, she had missed out on things mothers tell daughters about who to date, who not to date, what to look for in boys and what to avoid. Basically, "women's business", which is somewhat different from meeting up with your girlfriends for a drink.

So, we had girl time where I gave her the grandmother talk about boys, teaching her, as a relationships therapist, how to date, form and operate relationships and when to so say "No, thank you" and wave goodbye to unsuitable men. She was nervous about disclosure around her being trans, so I told her how I had dated men and women, some I told about being intersex and trans and some I did not. Our bodies are our own business and who we tell about them is our privilege, not anyone else's.

She started with what we called "mini dates" or "one-time" dates just to see if she liked the person. It was important that she made time to have those dates. She then had short affairs and to her surprise, she was having a really good time. The doubts about her transition disappeared along with the suicidal thoughts and she was even considering coming out to people.

Trans people are constantly bombarded with shame and guilt by society around being what we are. Samantha learned to own her own space like any woman, being beautiful, intelligent and worthy without apology.

Erick

A heterosexual male of 60, married for 40 years, with two adult professional children, Erick appeared to be the average guy. He had a highly successful printing business in which the family worked and was a part-time pastor at his church that was publicly extremely homophobic and transphobic. He lived in a small world based around the community of his work and religion where everyone knew everyone, or so they thought.

Erick had been a secret regular cross-dresser since he was 11 years old. He liked to wear female clothes, which sexually excited him. Six weeks previously, his wife had come home suddenly and found him dressed in clothes he kept in the attic. She was shocked and horrified, disclosing to their children and a church elder. A family meeting was called, which was basically like a court hearing, where he was given the ultimatum to cease the activity or his wife would divorce him and the church would ex-communicate him.

He managed to stop dressing for two weeks and then gave in to his urges. When I initially saw him, he had severe bruising of the face and was limping. Horrified at his perceived future prospects, he had driven his car into a tree to try and kill himself, but the car was expensive with all the safety features imaginable and it came off worse than he did.

Erick had no idea what he wanted from therapy, only that I was a sex and gender specialist and he saw it as a space where he could talk his situation through and I would not be shocked. He had never disclosed his cross-dressing to his wife when they got married so he had been deceiving her for 40 years and was not really surprised she was angry. The only way forward for him, he thought, was to stop cross-dressing.

While I said I was quite happy to help him, I made it clear that I was not going to buy into the restricted options he was framing for himself and me as a therapist, which was stopping dressing or fail. I explained that, from where I was sitting, it appeared that his whole life had been built around restricted options, which was why he was now sitting in my therapy chair: a marriage based on the missionary position, a prescriptive religion that told him how to live and a threatening family that told him it was their way or no way. He had built his own prison and then was upset when he was locked inside.

It was clear that after secretly dressing weekly for 49 years that he was unlikely to suddenly stop. So, what other options could there be? He was definitely clear that he did not want to split up with his wife who he loved very much. She was now seeing a church counsellor, no longer going to the business daily, refused to discuss their relationship and was virtually not speaking to him.

I explained to him the last thing you do is chase an angry person when they need space to think through their situation. He agreed they both needed time and space to explore the world outside their own community. He took an apartment next to the business for a year, moved in, resigned as a pastor at the church and attended therapy every week.

In therapy, he also owned that he enjoyed the comfort of dressing as female, which was a long way from the central patriarchal figure he had been acting out in his community. The suicide thoughts subsided and he saw that he did have other options and ways he could live his life. He discovered the world was indeed bigger than his own personal model of life. After six months, he was reunited with his wife and she agreed for him to have his own private sex life as she was no longer interested in sex. There was no longer a desire to end his life.

What Erick experienced was the perception of limited options and living from a place of fear. When his world was expanded outside the prison he had built for himself, there were better options than suicide.

First-Person Accounts of Life Over Suicide

Conor

It was only when I was an adult that I found out my parents took me to a psychiatrist when I was two years old because I was far from what my mother thought little girls should be. Always rough and tough, I was much more at home with the boys. I had no words for what I was in those days. I'd never heard of words like "transition" or "reassignment" or "realignment surgery".

I remember coming into my teenage years feeling I was male but convinced people would think I was crazy if I told them, so I buried those feelings for many years. My mother hated how I was but my dad accepted everything about me. The battles between my mother and I were so traumatic to me that I still suffer from complex PTSD today. Some members of my family still insist on referring to me as female and use the name I used to be called, so I have to limit contact with them so I am not triggered.

To bury those feelings, I started taking heroin and drinking at 13, running away from home, stealing cars and getting brought back home by the police. I was so self-destructive. When I was taken to court at 14 my mother didn't want me home so I lived at my best friend's house with his family. I was among the boys, which made life more tolerable.

I remember I'd pick fights with the biggest guys I could find, hoping it would end my life and I could check out, so I was definitely trying suicide by my actions. The heroin and self-destructive alcohol-taking lasted for a good 15 years until one day I was fixing-up and just thought, "What the hell am I doing? I'm killing myself". So, I went into a program to stop the addictions and got clean and sober.

I took a welfare course and started helping young people and getting involved in political justice and equal rights campaigns. It was a turning point for me because spending time trying to help others rather than just myself, I think saved my life.

I tried to fit into the lesbian community but something was always missing. There were good relationships and bad ones, people who expected me to be one particular thing and women who just saw me as a person, regardless of my sex or gender.

I didn't meet a trans guy who had transitioned until I was in my forties. In the lesbian community in those days there were many women who were anti-trans. When I came out and started to transition there were lesbians who told me I was doing the wrong thing and had trouble accepting me.

Now me and my beautiful dog live in a peaceful place and are supported by many good people. We don't all agree on everything but I've learnt to get along in a way that doesn't trigger my PTSD as much anymore. The fact that I've met so many nice, kind, friendly people over the years with no personal agenda, who accept me for the man I am made my life complete.

So, for me, choosing life over self-destruction came about by surrounding myself with accepting, loving people.

Katherine

I transitioned in 1990 when I was 18. Life was very difficult in those days especially for transgender people. There were many suicides within our community because there was no support or sense of community. Surviving was the main concern for us all in a world that rejected the very idea of the humanity of gender-diverse people.

Imagine being in a world where employment was refused to you, your family cut ties with you, society rejected the essence of your identity, and mainstream spirituality condemned you to Hell because you were born.

This life of isolation sent many gender-diverse people to end their lives all too soon. It was a "dog eat dog" world where trans people would also bully each other to feel self-worth about themselves. People can be cruel when they are jealous, insecure or feel powerless.

I too felt that isolation and damnation and wanted to die. I too thought I had nothing to live for. My strong Christian beliefs stopped me from ending my life, but I wanted to die, especially when the shadows of depression descended upon me when I turned 21. I had reached a milestone and nobody celebrated. I could not see an end to the discrimination and I had no emotional support from family or community.

My deep-rooted stubbornness gave me the strength to wade through while many others who transitioned at the same time began to take their own lives. I would estimate that only

10% of the transgender women I knew in 1990 are still alive. Not all of them committed suicide. Some of them accidentally overdosed on drugs and others were murdered or died from HIV and organ failure.

Nowadays, I am well-loved and respected within my community and by my peers. Looking from the outside my life would probably be described as blessed. But the real triumph of my story is I survived three decades. It is a life that I created for myself. I created my own employment as a gender diversity consultant, my own networks and I created my own niche in the world.

There was no destiny already waiting for me created by others. I would not have known this if I had ended my life at 21. I am so very blessed to have survived.

Happiness is a transient and temporary emotion. It is as changeable as the weather. I have learnt it is an impossible rainbow to chase. I have also learnt that contentment gives me the strength to carry on with life.

I have found contentment to be my constant companion to see me through; whether happy, sad, angry or chilled, I am always content—because I am Katherine, and my pronoun is SHE.

Sean

I was four years old when I told my mom that I wanted to be a boy. The funny thing is, I cannot remember telling her. She told me in early 2017 this bit of information and I was completely floored. I was speechless and scared.

I came out for the first time when I was 24 years old and I had just moved from South Africa to Australia and then again in 2017 as a female-to-male trans man (FtM).

Of course, the second time around had to be the year I turned 40. My brain had clearly done a great job at burying the truth of how I really felt, although my body had other ideas of how to manage all these buried treasures.

My entire life feels like a form of rebellion, every painful memory seems like a form of rebellion: the crying, the self-harm that no one knew of, the darkness and even the moments of light.

My physical self always had a problem with living. I have woken up every day of my life for the last 37 years hoping that "Today will be the day I feel better. Today will be the day I have a breakthrough".

I would get ready for work or go out to do mundane chores and within minutes the thought of death would cross my mind. I have considered so many avenues to hurt myself but as a registered nurse I learned that the risk of something going terribly wrong is just too high.

I was driving home one day from university in early 2017 and I was crying my eyes out. I came to a red light and I said out loud to myself, "You have a choice: death or testosterone—what is it going to be?"

I have been on testosterone for one year and a few months now and I am taking my anti-depressants religiously. I have stopped drinking because I have a PhD in music to finish. I have poems to write, music to record and perform, motivational speaking and communication masterclasses.

I have a partner who is a light in my life. My animals are awesome creatures who love me unconditionally and I don't want to leave them or my partner. I need them, and they need me.

Some days are better than others, but I keep going. No one else can make the music I make, no one else can bring my view on life and its secrets to the world but me. This is why I try to stick around. I have a story to tell and others to help.

Remember, you are not alone. Don't hide your feelings. Let them out in a safe place, and reach out for help, even if it means reaching out to strangers. Sometimes it is the strangers who make a world of difference. It makes the pain more bearable and facing life every day can become an inspiration for someone else.

Tracie (author of this book)

As an intersex, transexed child and young teenager born into poverty in the 1950s and 1960s in the north of England in the UK, I found the world very hostile. I was originally diagnosed as transsexual but as time passed it became obvious I had mild Androgyn Insensitivity Syndrome as my body did not masculinise properly and I was hypogonadal. My family were uneducated and rejected me. The health professionals who were supposed to be looking after me were negligent and abusive, treating my condition as a maladjusted behavioural issue. The prospect of a happy future looked very bleak indeed.

I attempted suicide more than once in my teenage years. I also suffered Post-Traumatic Stress Disorder in 2012, triggered by the abuse I encountered as a child, which made me think about suicide again.

The thing is, though, that overall life turned out pretty amazing. The people I have met and loved over the course of my life to date have inspired me to take charge of my own life and not rely solely upon the kindness of strangers.

Yes, life can be brutal at times and yes, being intersex and transexed has been very difficult at times over the years. Even now today, we still have to battle to have equal and fair treatment, but life has taught me it is not just about me being happy but about helping others be happy as well, whether they come from a SGD group or not.

The bleak times and dark night of the soul really can give way to wonderful life experiences and meeting incredibly kind and loving people when I myself make that happen. I have to reach beyond the fact that I was born intersex and transexed and find the champion within myself every day of my life. There is no free day when I can abandon my own self-care and loving and fall into the illusion the world is bad because I was born into a disadvantaged group of people.

So, choosing life over suicide has been a good choice for

me. If I think about the incredible experiences I have had, I realise that if suicide had been successful for me, I would have missed all those good times.

The friends I still have today, 50 years later, my darling wife, the people I adopted as my family, the friends I made fighting for civil rights and the kind folks who were nice to me just because they could be, all came into my life because I allowed them into my life and my heart.

I can tell you that life can get better when you put your mind to making that happen. Reach out and talk to people. Ask them for help. Take power for yourself and change some things so your life goes in another direction. Yes, sometimes it has to be big changes and sometimes small changes will make things happen.

During my life, people tried to stop me living as female, fired me from jobs because of what I am and a whole host of other horrific things happened to me, including physical and sexual assaults.

Don't let other people and disasters define you, but let them be an opportunity for you to make yourself stronger. Look for new opportunities and take action to make a good life for yourself, no matter what your circumstances are.

Choose what you are going to do to make life the better option over suicide and then do that again and again.

Bayne

I'm in a lot of official high-risk categories for suicidal ideation. Not just because I'm trans, but also being Goth and long-term disabled with Myalgic Encephalomyelitis (ME)/Chronic Fatigue Syndrome (CFS). I might also be autistic according to my autistic friends and though that's not officially diagnosed, I think it's not unlikely.

In my teens while facing a lot of bullying and struggling to repress my transness, I did have thoughts of suicide but they went away as I went into adulthood. When I came out, about to transition a decade and a half ago, suicidal thoughts did come back again. I guess it was because there were several things happening in my life at that time.

I can't really pinpoint a precise singular cause of the suicidal thoughts and feelings; some may be common and some not uncommon. I'd had a romantic disappointment but that happens to lots of people. I had issues with my disability, and its impact on my life compared to that of my less disabled and abled friends was getting to me. Again, that too wasn't particularly unusual. My disability has its emotional impact as it does for many of us. Still, something about that particular moment in time got to me unconsciously. I found myself feeling a sudden urge to end my life and it alarmed and frightened me.

My immediate response was very much to defy this urge. I proactively reached out to friends and made sure I wasn't alone. The dominant thoughts in my mind in response to these feelings was that throughout my life people had tried to stop me being me and I wouldn't surrender.

Being bullied as a child and teen tried to make me conform to the gender stereotypes of my assigned birth sex, to conform to male socially acceptable interests and supposed norms, like sport that I wasn't interested in. There was pressure to surrender or give up my geeky interests, hide my curiosity and love of books and the like. I experienced hostility from religious peers and adults who were determined that I share their beliefs and way of living, making who and what I was supposedly wrong.

All the standing up for myself led me, when I finally came to terms with being trans, to engage online and in-person in activism too. So, I fought prejudice as an adult the same way I'd fought the bullies, with reason and evidence and a fierce determination to be me and to stand up for myself and for others.

I was confused by these suicidal feelings that had come up. And I still am, even though they are now long gone.

Envy I suspect was part of it and grief over not being able to live my life with the automatic privileges that come so easily to many. And certainly, during the time I was struggling, the suicidal thoughts and feelings dredging up, exacerbating and exaggerating all the issues and struggles I'd ever had. My dysphoria was up with a vengeance, my hopes for the future felt hollow and impossible, and things that gave me strength and joy seemed empty or made me feel worse. I was suddenly filled with despondency.

But, if I gave in to those suicidal thoughts and feelings, it would mean all those bullies had won. They wanted me to be gone. They did not want me to be making a difference in the world or to be the difference in the world. That, I made up my mind, I would not allow. I would not make or allow all the effort and defiance I had mustered in my life, that had saved me, to be wasted. No, I would not let the bullies win.

The worst was over after about a couple weeks of spending as much time with friends as I could. That good and wholesome human connection fed me and helped me feel valid again. The trailing edges of the suicidal thoughts lasted another month I think, getting less and less with time. It's been over half a decade now and those thoughts and feelings of suicide have not returned. Sure, I struggle with life at times, but I am struggling for life, not against it.

Chapter 14:
Community-Based Model for Suicide Prevention

One of the things that became clear during the research for this project is that, despite the good intentions of those involved in setting up government-funded agencies to deal with suicide in people from SGD groups, they typically have limited capacity to service SGD groups. Many people who need help do not reach out to or cannot access those services, there may not be services in their area, or those services do not target those client groups well.

In 1979, Dr Paul McHugh closed the Johns Hopkins gender identity services in the US, shutting off the ability for patients to transition. It took four decades for his destructive work to be undone and the services to be resumed. He was quoted in the *Washington Post* as saying, "I'm not against transgender people but such help should be psychiatric rather than surgical" (Nutt, 2017).

The Charing Cross Gender Identity Clinic, UK, is so underfunded by the government that it takes three years to get into the program (Marsh, 2019). The longest wait time of five years in the UK NHS government clinics was 1,133 days in Nottingham. As a result, many patients end up taking non-prescribed hormones, putting themselves at risk of medical complications. The frustration of that wait clearly heightens the risk of suicide in some people.

In Africa, many countries persecute trans people even though there had previously been social spaces for gender diverse persons (Jobson et al., 2012). This means they are unable to access clinical help as in many places no such clinics exist and very little research has been carried out. Trans and intersex people are often classified as being homosexual, cursed and possessed by demons and pushed to the margins of society where there is absolutely no government help for them at all.

Under the present oppressive Putin regime in Russia, Dr Dmitri Isaev's gender clinic is not advertised, the location is kept secret and the phone number is not available (Patina, 2017). The Saint Petersburg location is hidden from public view for fear of intimidation. In Russia in general, treatment is not available and people who are from SGD groups are often prone to attacks and violence.

In developing countries like India, Pakistan and many others, there is little government-funded help for the health of trans groups; this is also the case in many rural areas (Safer et al., 2017). Healthcare professionals are not generally well trained in intersex medicine, clinics do not exist and governments may be oppressive towards these groups. Since they are not high-profile groups, governments assume they have few special needs.

When governments, politicians, policymakers, local authorities, funding, laws, health management and health practitioners change, the service can be withdrawn and disappear, even in developed countries. This leaves members of the SGD groups without support, isolated, disadvantaged, with increased mental health issues and more prone to suicide.

A further factor is that, in general, government-run ventures can often be ineffective and bogged down with endless bureaucracy that actually hinders the quality of healthcare. Administration generally takes up a large part of any allocated budget and practitioners are constantly under pressure to cut services and reduce costs. This can leave clients without adequate responses when faced with suicidal thoughts and actions.

The research quoted clearly shows elevated levels of bullying, violence, victimisation and harassment of SGD groups in both developed and developing countries. This happens regardless of the presence or absence of laws protecting these groups, leading to a high level of suicide risk.

The same is true when such services are married with services for gay, lesbian, bisexual and queer groups. In speaking to many people who have issues with their sex or gender, they stated they did do not feel comfortable accessing gay health services because they felt their issues were not understood or subsumed to queer politics. They saw the issues being facilitated in those spaces around sexuality when their issues were generally around sex or gender. For those of us who practise as mental health professionals in this field, we hear that many clients have never sought gay health services and do not wish to when having issues with their sex and gender.

Another clear fact when analysing the research was that despite people from SGD groups having access to professional medical and mental health services, they often seemed to be unable to reach out to those professionals when they are suicidal. They frequently do not feel connected to them or have the level of trust in those professionals that would give them sufficient confidence to reach out for help.

The conclusion can only be that government services are required and do help but what is equally as important is the need for community voluntary groups. People from the same or similar SGD groups often have a greater understanding of the issues that people from SGD groups face on a day-to-day basis that may drive them to suicide.

Modern state health systems are based on four principles: disease control, allopathic preference, evidence-based medicine and minimum cost. This reductionist and minimalist approach is plainly not working when suicidal thought patterns can be recorded as up to 60% in SGD populations.

We need a radical change in the way we approach the risk of suicide in SGD groups.

We need to take lessons from those who have come before us: like Alice Purnell (Le Duc, 2011) who helped start the Beaumont Society, Gender Trust and Gendy's Network in the UK; Roberta Perkins who started the Gender Centre in Australia (Anderson, 2018); Stephen Whittle who helped found the UK FTM network (Whittle, 2018); Crystal LaBeija who started the New York ball scene for African-American and Latina queens after encountering racism on the drag scene (Simon, 1968); and Mani Bruce Mitchell who worked in the intersex and queer spaces in New Zealand (Being Intersex, 2012). Their work clearly indicates that community associations save lives.

The film *Paris is Burning* demonstrates how the New York ball scene supported SGD street people and gay people who had largely been rejected by society (Livingston, 1990). It is the perfect fly-on-the-wall view of how the disenfranchised co-supported each other and is a classic example of community support due to community need. The house system that developed allowed isolated SGD people to join families of choice who watched out for them and their fragility in a hostile society.

There were, of course, many before these people from SGD groups who created safe spaces, working silently and often in secret for fear of persecution, to support people who struggled with suicide. They supported and befriended people through their darkest hours. These were people from SGD groups to whom the distressed could go if they were in trouble and needed help. There was no differentiation between whether they were intersex, transexual, transgender or androgynous; a hand of help would still be extended.

While not-for-profit organisations often fill some of the supportive roles, again they are subject to funding and staffing issues. If you have limited funds and staff, there are restrictions on what you can provide, what you can say and how you might be able to help people. Government-run or funded institutions can restrict the kind of outreach that can be offered by buddy systems, elders or young people's networks. They are often bound and constricted by bureaucratic dogma.

One way forward may be to change the approach of only funding government services and NGOs by funding more community-based groups. This would require governments to take a radically different approach to the health and mental health of this population. It would need government to focus funds on community groups and not just highly-qualified professionals who get the job because of their qualifications but may have little understanding of the client group or their life circumstances.

We can see how this works when we look at the trans coffee workers of Colombia who work picking coffee. Colombia is one of the most conservative Catholic and transphobic countries in the world and at least 300 people from LGBT groups had been murdered between 2017 to 2018 (Channel 4, 2019). The coffee workers gained employment and respect in their local area by being a contributing part of the workforce. Their association together helps them stay safe and give mutual support to each other to make their lives meaningful. It also gives them support in the local community because they are part of the spending community in the local economy.

SGD community groups must step out of their prejudices and segregation. Anyone who has a sex and gender difference can experience levels of prejudice, harassment, violence, discrimination and legal obfuscation. This discrimination, at times, is also by government laws and agencies. Community initiators and leaders must let go of their fears of other subgroups and focus on the job of helping people. It is not enough just to have a public voice as it also needs to be backed up by that community work. As SGD groups, we need to focus on our commonalities, not on our differences.

At SAGE Australia, we have always campaigned for the rights of all SGD groups and have not allowed ourselves to be drawn into the territory wars that take place between trans and intersex or trans and cross-dressers or femme drag queens or butch dykes who do or do not transition. Our members and campaigners are and have been from various spectrums of sex and gender diversity.

Buddies for Suicide Watch

In the 1980s as the AIDS crisis took off, we developed a scheme of voluntary buddying (Bressan, 1985). We would pair up with people who were experiencing full-blown AIDS to help them through their experience. We would visit them at home, in hospices, talk to them on the telephone, spend time with them, help them with their shopping and basically befriend them. It was very successful as a community exercise to bridge the gap between what health professionals could do for them and what they needed as human beings. Of course, many of those people died, as medical solutions were not advanced in those days, but the work we did improved the quality of their lives and even in the case of death.

People are at high risk days before a suicide attempt but often do not know where to reach out for help. The 28 days after a suicide attempt are probably the highest risk of further suicide. The depression, sense of hopelessness and reasons for suicide may still be prominent in the person's mind. Having a buddy who speaks to them for say 15 minutes by telephone every day can make all the difference in offering support. Someone who is genuinely interested in them, can listen, reassure, support, encourage and give them information for 15 minutes every day for 28 days can help them get past a suicide or post-suicide crisis period and get back on their feet.

In the case of Alexandra Greenway, a trans woman who had a degree in psychology and took her own life in Bristol in the UK in 2020, she had been waiting a month for help with suicide prevention. She was troubled with mental health issues and had attempted suicide. A psychiatrist had said that she would benefit from therapy, but no one contacted her. Greenway's mother said that previous staff who had helped her said they had focused on her issues at work rather than stress around her managing being trans (Morris, 2020). We can see from this case that intellect does not preclude SGD minority stress.

Even in modern healthcare systems, staff are overstretched and people fall through the cracks, not getting the care they need as fast as they need it in response to the threat of suicide. Also, professionals who are not from SGD groups often do not understand SGD stress. If Greenway had a suicide prevention buddy telephone call every day over that month, this could have supported her sufficiently to have saved her life.

The buddy does not take the place of the health professionals but instead helps feed the human need for contact and validation. Voluntary buddies can undergo a short training so they can remain objective in order to best help the person. They can also alert professionals and relatives if the client appears to go back into the suicide high-risk category.

The Use of Elders

In traditional societies, elders have an honoured, respected place of wisdom and serve as counsellors and helpers in their communities. This is none so prevalent as in Australian Aboriginal and Torres Strait Islander People for whom such elders are known as "Aunties" and "Uncles" (Huggins & Huggins, 2012).

Unfortunately, in Westernised societies, mature people have generally been relegated to the status of "old person", retired or past their use-by date. We have moved through a time when age has been seen as a handicap. We have become obsessed with efficiency, getting as much as you can for your money, health and safety over-caution, protecting jobs, and focusing on industrialisation, even within the caring professions. So, we have lost much of our elders' wisdom for healing, which has been replaced by scientific dogma that often has very poor evidence of its efficacy.

People from SGD groups can find themselves alone and living in isolation, which increases depression and thoughts of suicide. Perhaps they may have little or no contact with families and did not have children so life becomes isolated.

There are older people who have lived their lives in the sex and gender diverse space, have lived experience and have learnt many skills on how to survive and be happy. Would it not be wise for projects to marry the two communities together in an elder's program for people from SGD groups, creating a community and family of choice?

Here we would solve two problems and give each group a sense of belonging and connection. Many sex and gender diverse suicidal people who have been ostracised by families or society could experience validation and revivification of their sense of their own importance in the world.

Creating Young Communities

Industrialisation and post-industrialisation societies produce less and less actual human contact, with people retreating into technology and self-isolation, particularly with younger generations who grew up with digital technology. Therefore, when desperation and suicide become tempting, they are often misinformed by poor internet information and may be trolled online should they come out.

Each generation has its own language, understandings, gestalts and experiences, and they often do not translate into the values and experiences of other age groups, so communication can be vague or misunderstood. Some younger people can find older people boring and do not understand their cultural references.

Not only is it important for us to encourage younger people to create their own support networks but also to have them work with suicide rescue of people of their own age. They may also share many age-specific experiences and references that can be highly desirable in creating rapport with suicidal people from SGD groups of their own age.

They may need guidance and support at times in setting up networks, but they may be highly proficient at communicating electronically as technology was their ABCs of childhood. What we are also doing here is helping hand off the torch to future generations who will take over community care from the older generations in time.

Training Volunteers

Most trainings for volunteers or helplines are around two days long with a seven hours per day format. Many helplines are funded and employ professional counsellors who are paid, but here I propose also using unpaid volunteers from the SGD communities for projects working with minimal budgets and donations.

The reason for this is that when a project does not have to rely on official funding, it is not subject to funding withdrawal when political winds change. We have already seen the extreme difficulties in providing services by funded bodies that close or become inefficient or change, leaving clients in extreme distress.

Another reason to use unpaid volunteers from the SGD communities is that those people are often very dedicated to what they do. Even though some may not have a higher education, they can have street smarts and are highly skilled in life-coping skills and managing social spaces.

A perfect example of how effective this can be is seen in the Australian Aboriginal Tiwi Island sistergirls (Vice Asia, 2017). Some do not have family support, are not out in their community and there are no services available because they are so geographically remote. Having had high levels of suicide they have created sistergirl and brotherboy support networks where they befriend each other, give food and money and help each other when they are in need, including helping someone when they are suicidal.

Kindness and being present does not take a large amount of training, but those simple actions have profound effects on someone who is suicidal and can help pull them back from the abyss. These actions become more powerful when they are delivered by someone with whom you share commonalities like sex and gender differences.

Setting Up a Network

Setting up and sustaining a long-term voluntary network often generally comes down to the exhaustive efforts of a few people who are able to demonstrate dedication, stability, determination, consistency and tenacity. It is the day-to-day repetitious and dogmatic running of the administration that aids the functioning of such a network to provide those services.

Smith et al. (2021) offer a large collective of opinions and writings from 200 experts in over 70 countries on the theory and research of running voluntary operations, including not-for-profits.

Along the way, providers will encounter many detractors, critics and even those who seeks to undermine the network's actions for little or no reason. Running any voluntary network can at times be a thankless task, but the results of saving lives can be worth it in both the short- and long-term.

Volunteers need to be trained in suicide prevention during the two-day training and have a particular interest in the mental health area of work. Those volunteers can even be trainee mental health professionals who have experience working with SGD people. They do not necessarily need to be fully qualified to fill in when SGD volunteers are short as they are volunteer buddies. What administrators need to scan for is mental stability in volunteers. It is also pointless using volunteers who have absolutely no experience with or knowledge of people from SGD groups.

When helping clients, it may even be useful to direct them to particular volunteers who may be from the same SGD group so rapport can be built further. A client not having to explain themselves over and over again is a great relief. It also helps the client feel that they are not alone and that there are other people like them in the world.

Working in Groups

Five-person pods may be a good way to manage volunteers. One volunteer professional mental health worker manages a five-volunteer pod and runs a one-hour group supervision for that pod once a month. Plus, they are available for emergency supervision should a volunteer feel that they are out of their depth with a client.

Trainings need to include the practicum rehearsal of handling clients. It needs to give scope for the volunteer to understand what is expected of them, the limits of what they may do, the help they may offer, what they cannot offer and the help they themselves may receive to do the job.

Initial contact for clients' needs to come through the same port of call each time, with that administrator matching the client to a volunteer. The volunteer group also needs to observe client confidentiality in that a volunteer discussing a client with supervisors in supervision should use a pseudonym so the client's identity is protected. This can be difficult in small communities where others may recognise part of a client's story but, as much as possible, that confidentiality needs to be maintained, except in the case of imminent suicide.

The guidelines of conduct need to include not discussing anything about clients with anyone else, without the client's express written permission. This should apply to the volunteers the same as it applies to a health professional.

With volunteers helping clients with suicide ideations, it is important to contain the process. The volunteer is not a mental health professional and should not attempt therapy. Neither are they the client's friend because that would cause a loss of objectivity, which must always be maintained.

Contact with a buddy by telephone or electronic medium for 15 minutes for 28 days can change a person's life. It can help redirect the client's way of thinking, doing and where they are going in life. Setting that contact at the same time every day can also give stability to the client's situation.

Searching for Help

There is, however, a problem that volunteer groups face nowadays, which is Google. Traditionally support groups and charities have advertised their services in newspapers, magazines and through communities. They have traditionally been the mainstay safety net that took up the responsibility for help after state medicine reached its shortfall of service, which it constantly does.

Over the past ten years Google, which claims more than 92% of the global online searches, has heavily invested in pharmaceuticals along with its parent company Alphabet Inc. So, Google makes potentially billions of dollars a year from advertising the products of pharmaceutical companies. Much of this information is hard to find because technology companies edit what you see on the screen, but if you look, it is there.

At the same time Google became heavily invested in pharmaceuticals it changed its advertising policy to exclude self-help groups and private practitioners who are not using drugs from much of the advertising market (Google, 2021) (Koehn, 2019), especially in Australia. While Google says it is protecting the public from unethical help, it is in my opinion protecting its market share and manipulating access to help direct people towards drug-oriented solutions. Other tech companies have followed suit.

In other words, Google is shutting out the competition and at the moment governments are helpless and too afraid to regulate those trillion-dollar, profit-focused industries, although some have brought cases (Romm, 2020). Google has admitted manipulating access to news stories and politicians do not generally want to be their victim at the next election (Evershed, 2021). So, for the moment if you run a voluntary group, constantly SEOing your site is probably the best way to get before your potential client group, along with social media posting and media exposure rather than running ads.

Insuring Volunteers

Even if someone is a volunteer, an unpaid worker or working in a cluster of helping people, it is wise to have insurance whenever possible. When working with suicidal people, some will complete suicide, which may leave a volunteer in danger of being sued. No one may have done anything wrong and they may have been diligent in their duties, but nuisance lawsuits can be brought by relatives when they are in distress and trying to find someone to blame for the death.

Each country will have their different laws around legal settlements so it is important to thoroughly investigate what a policy may and may not cover. America and Canada are the most litigious countries and often subject to many unworthy lawsuits where volunteers could be ruined due to personal liability. Also, insurance companies often do not want to fight cases and are willing to settle out of court with no public declaration of liability. At times, insurance companies try to force the insured into admitting liability with a low pay-out to the plaintive.

Volunteers can be traumatised by a client's suicide as they are not trained health professionals and do not understand that suicide happens in the health industry despite the professional help people receive. So, at times, organisers run the risk of volunteers suing them for post-traumatic stress disorder.

Since claims may be genuine or bogus, it is important to limit financial losses to a bare minimum by having as comprehensive an insurance policy as possible for all involved. As the group needs to be run by a mental health practitioner, it may be possible to put counselling student volunteers on the practitioner's policy.

There are also policies specifically for volunteer workers that the volunteers can take out themselves. For instance, at the moment, the cost of such a policy in Australia is around AUD$300 per annum, but that may be much higher in America or Canada. It is also important that a client from outside the insured zone should not be facilitated, which would render the insurance invalid. Some policies, however, do cover multiple countries, sometimes with exemptions for America and Canada, if it is taken out outside those zones. North America and Canada can be included for a minimal extra cost in some policies.

Volunteers must be legally made fully aware of the realities and limitations of insurance during their training process. Each person has a responsibility to protect the network as much as protect the clients and volunteers so that as many clients as possible can be facilitated safely.

In setting up a buddy network, it is important to make it clear to the client that the 28 days is a one-time offer for buddy support. Buddy suicide networks would be ill-advised to take clients for longer or repetitively as that would go beyond the voluntary buddy paradigm and cross over into social work, for which volunteers are not qualified.

As the far-right prospers in parts of the world and SGD groups can become illegal, insurance may become null and void in some places. The provision of services may become illegal as public recognition and protection of SGD groups get rolled back by some governments, while in some places it was never in place. In March 2020, Hungary, under Prime Minister Viktor Orban, proposed a law to rescind all recognition of trans and intersex people, ceasing to allow them to change their birth certificates and documents (Knight & Gall, 2020). Under these circumstances, volunteers can be exposed to risks of persecution themselves so outreach work from other countries that share a common language may be the only option.

Linguistic and Cultural Diversity in Volunteers

It is also important to remember that using counselling students has benefits and drawbacks for such networks. They may seem easier to find and train but they may have little understanding of SGD issues and the circles and subcultures in which those clients move; and SGD groups do have subcultures.

Since many of us live in a cosmopolitan world, often in a metropolis, we may live in cultures with multiple languages and belief systems. It is impossible for us as individuals to understand all the gestalts, social dynamics and linguistic nuances that operate in the client's first language or culture. Co-opting volunteers from those cultures can go a long way to facilitating those client's needs as they have a greater understanding of the pressures and obstacles faced in the client's daily life.

In running a project, it is just as important to let those volunteers know their ethnic diversity is valued and send out regular communications to volunteers so they feel connected to the team.

The Pivotal Resetting of Service Provision

There is little doubt that the COVID-19 global pandemic affected service delivery to marginalised groups. As countries went into lockdown and isolation to control the spread of the virus, services ceased to be delivered to many SGD groups. Hormones became in short supply, surgeries were cancelled, mental health support was cut and many people were isolated on their own in lockdown for months, suffering profound depression.

Electronic communication, however, became paramount in much of the world. In China, it is impossible to communicate with the government unless you have a mobile telephone. People in the West turned to Facebook and other social media platforms to communicate with each other. Those who had avoided technology found themselves out of the loop and unable to navigate the system. As mobile sales initially went down, so did prices, so less-advantaged people could join the techno-local revolution. For many, however, that was not true as people lost their jobs and sources of income.

Social distancing for fear of virus contraction changed the way we communicated as human beings, not holding, hugging or standing close to people. It changed the way we delivered mental health support to people, whether in the private sector, charitable or government sectors. In wake of the crisis, at the time of writing, less help was available to SGD groups from government or healthcare system services.

To the extreme right-wing, the COVID-19 crisis became a great opportunity to marginalise SGD groups even more. Behind the panic of the spread of the virus, right-wing groups had specialised teams working out how they could use the pandemic to withdraw human rights from SGD groups of people. In Central Park, New York, which was hit hard by the virus, thousands of people died. Samaritan's Purse, an evangelical Christian group, set up a medical tent but publicly refused service to gay, trans and identified intersex people (Browning, 2020).

In Hungary, the right-wing attacked the rights of intersex and trans people to be recognised (Walker, 2020). In Uganda, homes of trans people, along with gay people, were raided and those living in homeless shelters were arrested just because of who they were, on the pretext of preventing the spread of COVID-19 (Ghoshal, 2020).

In Panama, to stop the spread of the virus, women were allowed out on one day and men on alternative days, and a trans woman was arrested for giving out food on the women's day (Ott, 2020). Poland's governing Law and Justice Party (PiS), backed by the Catholic church, attacked and denounced "LGBT ideology" and tried to eliminate rights for SGD groups (Poland is Australia's 'Logical Conclusion', 2020). In the UK, during COVID-19, the Equality Minster Liz Truss launched a proposed law change that those under 18 not be allowed to transition, against the advice of the medical establishment (Reid-Smith, 2020).

Whether you are a health professional managing a full caseload, or a manager or volunteer working on a buddy helpline, there is a need to monitor yourself for compassion fatigue. With all the good intentions in the world, we must remember as helpers that we are also human beings and must take care of our owns needs to be effective.

The Professional Quality of Life Measure 5 Self-Score Measure (ProQOL, 2020) is probably one of the most commonly-used indexes of compassion fatigue. Since suicide is a stressful field to work in, I recommend that practitioners take the time to self-examine. Managers, team leaders and supervisors are wise to require their staff and volunteers to regularly take the questionnaire, not only as a care procedure but also to reduce the liability of industrial action or lawsuits.

I started this book exposing you to the atrocities that people from SGD groups experience on day-to-day basis. You might have wanted to see that information as historical, but it is not. As you can now see, it is ongoing. It is cyclical according to the stage of the eternal fight between extreme conservatism and liberalism.

The reality is that these attacks on SGD groups of people will never cease. We will always be fighting for equal rights. When the news is quiet, ultra-conservative, politicians will seek to gain public attention by attacking soft target minorities like SGD groups. Delusional religious cults will make prognostications that SGD groups are possessed by the devil. When a disaster happens, some seeking attention will again look for minority groups to blame. This is not a conspiracy theory but simply human interaction.

Since the beginning of this research, however, a new factor has begun to be recognised. This is the breakdown of social order and democracy due to the influence of social media, which causes social polarisation and an increase in minority victimisation. The documentary drama *The Social Dilemma* (Orlowski, 2020) shows us how social media algorithms lead to interest groups only receiving news stories that reflect their digital footprint, meaning no two people get the same news.

This has created the Pizzagate effect (in 2016 thousands of people spread a false rumour about a US pizza restaurant being a front for a child sex ring) where false news leads to people taking action against targeted groups and individuals. This clearly happens when many SGD groups and people are targeted on the internet. Attacks incited by the far-right and religious groups based on falsely-created facts and information happen. During the COVID-19 crisis, and accompanying social paranoia and hysteria, many people from SGD groups felt more unsafe in their communities with higher levels of depression, isolation and at a greater risk of suicide. The effect will only increase as the ever-increasing, profit-driven technocracy promotes social division.

As you can see, people from SGD groups do not necessarily attempt suicide because they are having an existential crisis but because the environmental and social pressures upon them are so oppressive that they lose hope and can only see a bleak future for themselves.

The sheer cost of responding to the COVID-19 crisis has put governments into a massive borrowing mode, sending their balance sheets severely into the red. Businesses were destroyed and governments lost control of their economies, which meant they were forced to severely cut funds to minority services providing help to SGD groups, just the same as they cut costs for services to other minorities.

This is why self-help groups can once again become so important, particularly for the support of people who may feel suicidal. SGD groups and communities themselves need to step forward and be part of the solution for their members who are suicidal.

You can start a suicidal helpline on a shoestring budget and donations and run by volunteers. You may decide to avoid looking for government funding because it comes and goes. When organisations become dependent on it, they have to abide by a plethora of rules set up by people who do not know what the organisation does. When funding ceases, a funded-dependent group ceases to function. Also, quality of care audits are frequently disguised as political compliance protocols. If you set up a volunteer group, it may be worth exploring getting grants from government, corporations or charities and philanthropic donors, but always be careful that it does not constrain what you set out to achieve in the first place.

To those of you who are from SGD groups, I say to you, "We need to look after our own". We may be different in many ways, but if we are from these marginalised SGD groups, we need to step up and give back.

Government Bodies and NGOs Need to Work with Volunteer Groups

In this book, I have both praised and criticised the work that government organsitions, NGOs and employees do, but as physicist Stephen Hawkins said, "There is no science without critic".

During my research, many government-run bodies and

NGOs refused to circulate a call-out for participation in the research. Their excuses were, "You are not part of our organisation", "You do research differently from the way we approve", "We cannot work with voluntary groups, we are professionals". This is despite the fact that I had been working in the field since before many of the respondents were born, have previously published four books on the subject plus many articles and papers, have spoken at many professional conferences, ran a private practice for decades and have been active in the voluntary work and campaigning sector for SGD groups for 50 years.

The sad truth behind such responses is that when people get jobs, they defend their jobs against all kinds of what they perceive to be competition so they can pay their mortgages and continue to go on holiday. This attitude by health professionals does not serve SGD groups—ever.

What serves SGD groups of people, as a marginalised people, is that they can get the help they need from wherever it might be available; and that all kinds of organisations are willing to work together to serve the needs of these people, particularly when it comes to suicide prevention and rescue.

The dead do not care about politics

As SGD groups, we have had to fight for our rights individually and collectively and we have to fight to maintain them again and again. Fighting each other or health professionals fighting over who has the right to help and collect a pay cheque is counterproductive.

United we stand—divided we fall

So many of our community have lost their lives to suicide, not always because of their desperate need of highly-qualified professional help but instead due to the absence of someone taking the time to pay attention to them, a kind word, smile and a thimble of hope.

None of us are free unless we're all free

The Political Act of Helping SGD Groups
Helping SGD groups as a minority in a hostile environment is of itself a political act. My work began five decades ago when I had to operate in secret as a teenager, due to fears of my own personal safety.

Over the years, I have experienced attacks from other health professionals for being intersex and trans, harassment from the police and do-gooder zealots, the right-wing for being radical, the left-wing for being in private practice and appearing to them bourgeois and profiteering, fellow professionals who consider clients from SGD groups deranged who must be managed, fellow professionals for even working in the field, association regulators who wished to deregister me when I came out publicly as intersex and trans, relatives of clients who do not want the client to assert themselves, many of my own relatives who are ashamed that I am what I am, the media who try to sensationalise sex and gender diverse issues...and the list goes on. But I and many of my wonderful peers are still here.

When you work in the public sector and take government funds, you run the risk of being gagged on the political issues around SGD groups' human rights. When public sector workers become public political campaigners, they can be sanctioned, deselected from promotion and even fired. I am a political animal and SAGE is a political collective. Change can only occur when professionals and the public are prepared to stand up and be heard. Academia and clinical practice alone changes little and runs the risk of the most important conversations only being held behind closed and closeted privileged doors.

The advantage of a volunteer network is that it is not

subject to the constrictions of state oppression and the fear of people being fired from their jobs to be quietened, so members can speak out publicly about human SGD rights. The suicide of people from SGD groups is largely tied up with their imbibed inferior perceptions of themselves that have been influenced by an often hostile political environment.

Any supportive help for people from SGD groups who are suicidal can contribute towards their lives. All of us as helpers are valid in our own efforts, the time we spend, energy we bring, years we study and hours we work frequently beyond what is contractually required.

When we come from a place of fear we breed, teach and condone fear. Oppression is political; therefore we as healthcare professionals, carers and volunteers need to be political advocates for SGD groups. Only then are we practising the full art of healing.

References

Anderson, C. (2018). Remembering Roberta Perkins. *Overland*. Retrieved from https://overland.org. au/2018/11/remembering-roberta-perkins/

Being Intersex: 'I went from being my parents' son to a daughter' (2012, April 26). *NZ Herald*. Retrieved from https://www.nzherald.co.nz/lifestyle/being-intersex-i-went-from-being-my-parents-son-to-a-daughter/UZ5R7HSBBM4FMSIVIGPPXCEHGY/

Bressan, A. (1985). *Buddies* [Motion picture]. United States: Film and Video Workshop

Browning, B. (2020, March 31). Viciously anti-LGBTQ group runs Central Park tent hospital & forces volunteers to reject gay rights. *LGBTQ Nation*. Retrieved from https://www.lgbtqnation.com/2020/03/

viciously-anti-lgbtq-group-runs-central-park-tent-hospi-tal-forces-volunteers-reject-gay-rights/

Evershed, N. (2021, January 27). Important stories hidden in Google's 'experiment' blocking Australian news sites. *The Guardian.* Retrieved from https://www.theguardian.com/technology/2021/jan/28/important-stories-hidden-in-googles-experiment-blocking-australian-news-sites

Ghoshal, N. (2020, April 3). Uganda LGBT shelter residents arrested on COVID-19 pretext. *Human Rights Watch.* Retrieved from https://www.hrw.org/news/2020/04/03/uganda-lgbt-shelter-residents-arrested-covid-19-pretext

Google ads (advertising policy), 2021. Retrieved from https://support.google.com/adspolicy/answer/176031?hl=en-AU

Huggins, R., & Huggins, J. (2012). *Auntie Rita.* Aboriginal Studies Press.

Jobson, G., Theron, L., Kaggwa, J. & Kim, H. (2012). Trans-gender in Africa: Invisible, inaccessible, or ignored? *Sahara-J: Journal of Social Aspects of HIV/AIDS*, 9(3), 160–163. Retrieved from https://doi.org/10.1080/17290376.2012.743829

Koehn, E. (2019). 'Absolutely unacceptable': Business fury over Google ad policy. *The Sydney Morning Herald.* Retrieved from https://www.smh.com.au/business/small-business/absolutely-unacceptable-business-fury-over-google-ad-policy-20190814-p52gvy.html

Knight, K., & Gall, L. (2020, May 21). Hungary ends legal recognition for transgender and intersex people. *Human Rights Watch.* Retrieved from https://www.hrw.org/news/2020/05/21/hungary-ends-legal-recognition-transgender-and-intersex-people

Le Duc, F. (2011, December 31). New year honours for Brighton and Hove LGBT supporters. *Brighton & Hove News.* Retrieved from https://www.brightonandhovenews. org/2011/12/31/new-year-honours-for-brighton-and-hove-lgbt-supporters/12027/

Livingston, J. (1990). *Paris is burning* [Motion picture]. United States: Academy Entertainment

Marsh, S. (2019, November 20). Transgender people face years of waiting with NHS under strain. *The Guardian.* Retrieved from https://www.theguardian.com/society/2019/nov/20/transgender-people-face-years-of-waiting-with-nhs-under-strain

Morris, S. (2020, October 18). Bristol transgender woman who took own life felt fobbed off, family say. *The Guardian, UK.* Retrieved from https://www.theguardian.com/society/2020/oct/18/transgender-woman-who-took-own-life-felt-fobbed-off-by-bristol-mental-health-services

News. (2019). Meet Colombia's trans coffee pickers [Video file, Facebook]. *Channel 4.* Retrieved from https://www.facebook.com/Channel4News/videos/361128971105106/UzpfSTY2MjI5MzE5Mzg6MTAxNTY0ODc4ODA2N-jY5Mzk/

Nutt, A. E. (2017, April 6). Johns Hopkins psychiatrist sees hospital come full circle on transgender issues. *The Washington Post.* Retrieved from https://www.baltimoresun.com/health/bal-johns-hopkins-transgender-20170406-story.html

Orlowski, J. (2020). *The Social Dilemma Documentary-drama* [Motion picture]. United States: Film and Video Workshop.

Ott, H. (2020, April 10). Trans woman fined for violating Panama's gender-based coronavirus lockdown, rights group says. *CBS News*. Retrieved from https://www.cbsnews.com/news/trans-woman-fined-for-violating-panamas-gender-based-coronavirus-lockdown-rights-group-says-2020-04-10/

Patina, K. (2017, February 1). Russian doctor defies intimidation to authorise gender reassignment surgery. *The Guardian*. Retrieved from https://www.theguardian.com/society/2017/feb/01/russian-doctor-defies-intimidation-to-authorise-gender-reassignment-surgery

Poland is Australia's 'logical conclusion' of excluding LGBTQI people with religious discrimination bill. (2020, April 27). *Star Observer*. Retrieved from https://www.starobserver.com.au/features/human-rights/poland-is-australias-logical-conclusion-of-excluding-lgbtqi-people-with-religious-discrimination-bill/194800

PROQol. (2020). Retrieved from https://www.proqol.org/

Reid-Smith, T. (2020, April 23). UK launches unprecedented attack on trans rights, will ban transition before 18. *Gay Star News*. Retrieved from https://www.gaystarnews.com/article/uk-launches-unprecedented-attack-on-trans-rights-will-ban-transition-before-18/

Romm, T. (2020). Justice Department sues Google, alleging multiple violations of federal antitrust law. *The Washington Post*. Retrieved from https://www.washingtonpost.com/technology/2020/10/20/google-antitrust-doj-lawsuit/

Safer, J., Coleman, E., Feldman, J., Garofalo, R., Hembree, W., Radix, A. & Sevelius, J. (2017). Current Opinion in Endocrinology. *Diabetes & Obesity*, 23(2), 168–171. doi: 10.1097/MED.0000000000000227

Simon, F. (1968). *The queen*. [documentary]. Grove Press

Smith, D., Stebbins, A. & Grotz, J. (2021, February 19). *The Palgrave handbook of volunteering, civic participation, and nonprofit associations.* Palgrave McMillan

Vice Asia. (2018). Sistagals: Australia's Indigenous gay and trans communities [documentary]. Retrieved from https://www.youtube.com/watch?v=XReQrGyJXIE

Walker, S. (2020, April 3). Hungary seeks to end legal recognition of trans people amid Covid-19 crisis. *The Guardian.* Retrieved from https://www.theguardian.com/world/2020/apr/02/hungary-to-end-legal-recognition-of-trans-people-amid-covid-19-crisis

Whittle, S. (2020). *Lesbian, gay, bisexual, trans history month.* Retrieved from https://lgbtplushistorymonth.co.uk/2011/03/stephen-whittle/

Afterword

During this three-year project, much has changed and is still changing now. I had to step back from the research several times as SAGE members lobbied the Australian Government on different laws that proposed to diminish SGD rights. The Federal Labor Party dumped swaths of legal amendments for civil rights for SGD groups of people from its manifesto in order to court the religious vote at the next election.

Joe Biden succeeded Donald Trump as President of the United States and tried to reverse much of the legal and social damage that Trump did to SGD people's rights. The conservative states revolted, however, issuing a whole raft of laws at local level levels against SGD groups' rights.

The European Union declared itself an LGBTIQ Freedom Zone, trying to bring in line countries like Poland that had declared itself an LGBTIQ Free Zone. This is a collective of countries that Europe is unable to control that operates extreme right-wing and religious policies that oppress SGD groups.

The COVID-19 crisis left many disadvantaged people from SGD groups in poverty, with little to eat, unable to pay for rent or medical expenses, and jobless. Many of these are populations that will not recover a financial foothold in the next economic boom because they had hung on at the financial margins for years.

The United Nations continues to be ineffectual in amending civil rights for SGD groups. Many member countries simply choose to ignore resolutions, without any kind of penalties.

Therefore, the swing between the extreme right-wing and libertarians continues like an ever-rebounding pendulum becoming more violent as social media algorithms accelerate the divisions in society.

Caught in the middle of all this is the individual from a SGD group who is battling to survive, traumatised and, in many cases, experiencing suicidal thoughts. As groups, we have gone from being a media curiosity, fodder for sensationalist headlines and on to being a public enemy, as clickbait material.

This is a time of continual ongoing oppression and violence towards SGD groups. The traumas and anxieties that drive people from these groups towards suicide will not end soon, as these are caused by ongoing sexism and genderism.

We should not just be do-gooders as healing health professionals but warriors on behalf people from SGD groups. We are often their lifeline to wellbeing and survival.

In the face of this continual oppression more people are speaking up for SGD groups and people from those groups are standing up and being counted. From necessity springs hope eternal.

As the trans actress Dominique Jackson said in her acceptance speech for an award at the 23rd Human Rights Campaign National Dinner:

"Our foundation is human—not sex. It is not about saying to someone else, 'I accept you', or 'I tolerate you'. You do not have the power to accept or tolerate me. I take that from you. You will respect me."

Please help those from SGD groups who experience suicidation to recover the will to live and find joy in life. Remember, however, that when you have helped them, they will go back out into the world where, once again, they will suffer the onslaughts of prejudice, so above all teach them resilience.

Thank you for your attention.

Go save lives!

Resources

I have made the following documents available for you to use as a guide to create your own. You can access them at the URL provided below:

→ Short Suicide Questionnaire
→ Addiction Questionnaire
→ Sample Client Contract for Buddy Services
→ Sample Guidelines for Volunteers in Suicide Prevention Buddy Groups
→ Application Form to Become a Buddy
→ Assessment Criteria for Determining Suitability of Buddys
→ Daily Volunteer Report (which can be installed as a template in a CRM system)

Download these documents as PDFs and amend them for your own use from:

www.doctorok.com/sgdbookresources

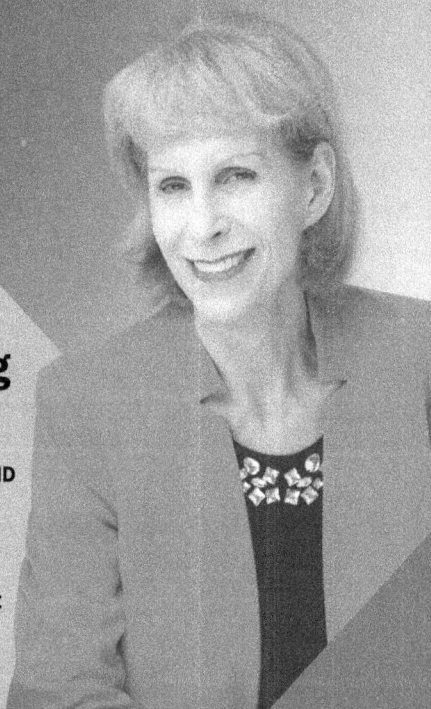
352

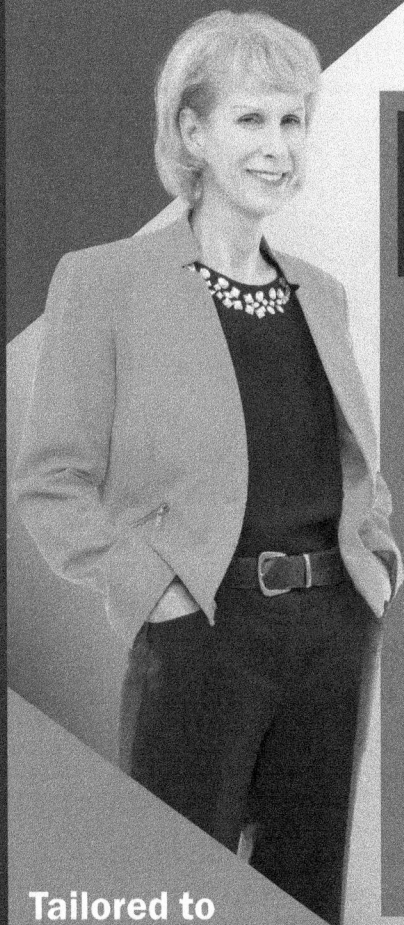

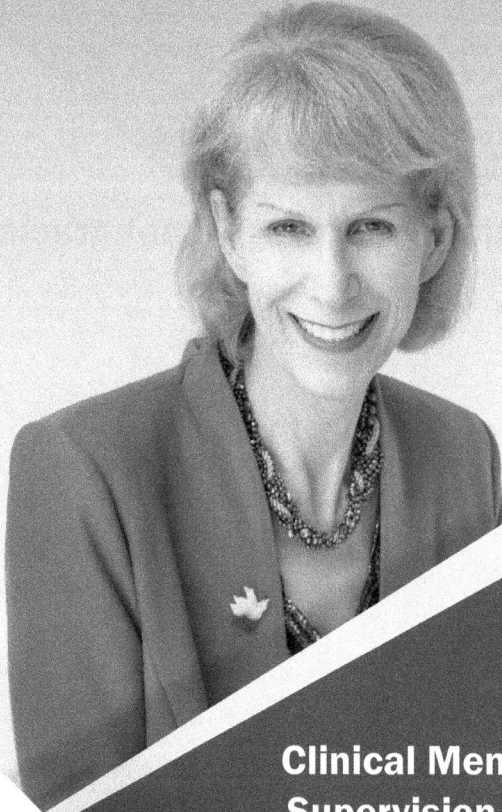